Conjuring *the* State

Pitt Latin American Series

Catherine M. Conaghan, Editor

Conjuring *the* State

Public Health Encounters in Highland Ecuador, 1910–1945

A. Kim Clark

University of Pittsburgh Press

Published by the University of Pittsburgh Press, Pittsburgh, Pa., 15260

Manufactured in the United States of America
Printed on acid-free paper
10 9 8 7 6 5 4 3 2 1

Cataloging-in-Publication data is available from the Library of Congress

ISBN 13: 978-0-8229-4782-0
ISBN 10: 0-8229-4782-X

Cover art: Plague encounters in highland Ecuador: Nisag, Chimborazo, 1929.
From *Public Health Reports* 45, no. 36 (September 5, 1930).
Cover design: Melissa Dias-Mandoly

To Juliana, Marisol, and Alejandro, who have been living with this project—or living with me living with this project—for their whole lives. They are the best kind of distraction and inspiration.

Contents

Acknowledgments

In 1991, while carrying out local archival research in Alausí for my doctoral dissertation on the history, culture, and political economy of the Ecuadorian railway project, to my surprise I came across documents about a bubonic plague outbreak in the area. Not only was I unaware of the third pandemic of plague that reached the Americas at the turn of the twentieth century, but I also had no idea at the time that there continued to be a reservoir of plague just up the mountains from the town of Alausí. While I wrote briefly about plague in the book that resulted from my PhD research, *The Redemptive Work: Railway and Nation in Ecuador, 1895–1930*, the epidemic continued to pique my curiosity enough to lead me to the archives of the Museo Nacional de Medicina in Quito during a postdoctoral project in 1993 and through numerous subsequent research trips. The documentation I found there revealing the everyday practices of the Public Health Service opened up new lines of inquiry for me, stimulating not only questions about the social history of medical and public health practices in Ecuador but also new questions informed by the anthropology of the state. It took me many years to think through which of several possible stories I wanted to tell from this fascinating material and to shape this book. Along the circuitous route to this outcome, I wove another narrative from portions of this broader archival material in what I consider to be this book's companion volume, *Gender, State, and Medicine in Highland Ecuador: Modernizing Women, Modernizing the State, 1895–1950*—which, in an early incarnation, began as a chapter of this book until it substantially outgrew its origins.

The research on which this book draws was carried out in several Ecuadorian archives over an extended period of time. I would especially like to thank the wonderful staff at the Museo Nacional de Medicina (housing the Archivo del Servicio de Sanidad as well as the Archivo de la Asistencia Pública and the Archivo del Hospital Civil San Juan de Dios) and the staff at the Archivo General de la Universidad Central. As suggested, it was also inspired by my first archival research in the Archivo de la Jefatura Política de Alausí and the Archivo del Consejo Municipal de Alausí. Friends and colleagues in Quito discussed these materials with me over many years: Rocío Bedón, Guillermo Bustos, Valeria Coronel, Antonio Crespo, Patricia de la Torre, Sonia Fernández, Ana María Goetschel, Eduardo Kingman Garcés, Dr. Eduardo Luna Yépez, María (Maruja) Martínez de Suárez, Fabiola Montúfar, Elena Noboa, Pablo Ospina, Mercedes Prieto, Guadalupe Soasti, and Luis Suárez Martínez. Feedback from colleagues and friends on conference presentations and drafts of chapters or chapter sections over the last two decades is much appreciated: my thanks to Tracey Adams, Michiel Baud, Marc Becker, Juanita de Barros, Greg Beckett, David Carey Jr., Paulo Drinot, Chris Krupa, Raúl Necochea, David Nugent, Erin O'Connor, Steve Palmer, Jadwiga Pieper Mooney, Liz Roberts, Veronica Schild, Alan Smart, Jay Stock, Adam Warren, and Eliza Williamson. I have been thinking and talking through this material for so long that I have undoubtedly overlooked some conversations that influenced my thinking. Friends in the Anthropology Department at Western University heard versions of these materials over many years, sometimes prompting them to ask, "Yes, but is the *entire* book about bubonic plague?!" I have been exceptionally lucky to have departmental colleagues who have been so supportive in so many areas of my work and life.

Another kind of support came from my Classical Studies colleague Kelly Olson, who suggested that despite—or perhaps because of—my role as department chair, I needed a partner with whom I would agree to meet on a weekly basis to write (and sometimes to "write"). Her insistence that we had an obligation to each other to sit together with our laptops, away from the chair's office, to write on a regular schedule helped me to bring this project to completion, despite many distractions. This morphed into a university-wide faculty writing support program led by Kelly and Emily Ansari. During my post-chair pandemic research leave, I found new writing companions online with the Anthro Co-Write group on Discord, organized by Laurie Denyer Willis. It was truly a joy to hop on at scheduled times or random hours of the day or night and find someone on another coast or another continent who was also looking for company to do some cowriting—in thanks, I am sending out emoji hearts and gifs of cats typing and babies cheering to all the shifting members of this merry band!

I am grateful for the productive conversations about these materials at two research workshops which came at key moments for imagining the shape of this book's larger argument. Paulo Drinot and Lawrence Brown gave me the opportunity to engage with historians of medicine working elsewhere in Latin America and the Caribbean at a wonderful workshop in Manchester in September 2009. Chris Krupa and David Nugent, in turn, brought together a stimulating group of anthropologists and historians at a conference in Quito on Off-Centered States: State Formation and Deformation in the Andes in May 2010. These two groups of colleagues each challenged me to address different kinds of scholarly questions in my writing and to deepen and extend my analysis in new directions. As the writing process advanced, the opportunity to exchange book manuscripts with Paulo Drinot and to workshop them together in London, UK, in February 2019 was invaluable. Special thanks to Paulo for uttering the words, "If this is history of public health, then why wouldn't you . . ." (among many other constructive comments), which clarified for me that only incidentally was I thinking of this as a history of public health, and that I needed to be much clearer about its framing. Thanks also for his excellent advice to find a book title that captured the book's argument and not just its content. The discovery that David Carey Jr. was doing related work from a comparative perspective led to another opportunity to workshop our respective book manuscripts in 2020, which among other productive outcomes helped me to identify some distinctive elements of this project. I am also grateful to the two sets of reviewers for the press who provided feedback on my analysis, first as an early draft and then a much more polished one. I came to learn that Ernesto Capello was one of the early reviewers, providing a generously worded nudge to deepen my analysis (and redeeming the label Reviewer 2). And in round two, I could hear Chris Krupa's voice echoing in my head as I read a set of comments, sounding so much like that time he said to me in person, "This is good . . . but I think you can do more." Thanks to Ernie, Chris, and the two other anonymous reviewers for their encouragement, support, and insistence that I could push my analysis further. Peer review at its best.

Given that this book draws on research carried out across a variety of projects over three decades, various funding agencies supported research that contributed to it. I am grateful for generous funding from Associated Medical Services, Toronto (for three grants); the Wenner-Gren Foundation for Anthropological Research, New York (for two grants); the Social Sciences and Humanities Research Council of Canada (for doctoral and postdoctoral fellowships that set me on the path to discover these new interests); and the University of Western Ontario (for an International Research Award as well as support from the Agnes Cole Dark Fund within the Faculty of Social Science). Finally, it was an honor to be named a Faculty Scholar for Social Science for the period

2015–2017, and in material terms that gave me the resources to complete the writing process, including support for additional travel to discuss the manuscript with colleagues. As a scholar who has built her research through relatively small grants of $5,000–$10,000, I am grateful for these programs that were scaled to my modest needs.

Special thanks to two people who made an extra effort to help me gather and decipher the enrollment records of the Faculty of Medicine at Quito's Central University, which helped me understand the practitioners who populate this book. On one of our briefer trips to Ecuador, my daughter Juliana (aged twelve at the time) brought her digital photography skills to my work to gather what would otherwise have been weeks' worth of material in two days. And my PhD student Christian Español spent long hours (longer than either of us expected) organizing a database of those enrollment records. It was stimulating to discuss this material with him as he considered state formation in Venezuela. Another doctoral student, Jordan Levy, was analyzing his research materials on Honduran teachers as I worked through my data on Ecuadorian public health physicians, leading to many productive conversations about state agents. Since then, the opportunity to supervise two more doctoral students working on the anthropology of the state in Latin America—Beatriz Juárez and Luis Meléndez—has helped me to think more deeply about my own research. Most recently, Natalia Parra (to whom I owe thanks for her work organizing some of the scattered archival information about plague cases) and Daniela Barba have joined this group of doctoral students exploring political anthropology in and of Latin America. I have learned a great deal from thinking alongside my graduate students as we explore these shared research interests. As I was finishing final revisions to this manuscript, it was a special treat to teach a graduate seminar on the anthropology of the state to a group of MA and PhD students from across the subfields of anthropology in fall 2021; I thank them for so many stimulating discussions.

It continues to be a pleasure to work with the University of Pittsburgh Press and the Pitt Latin American Series, edited by Catherine Conaghan. I again had a wonderful experience with them, starting with Josh Shanholtzer's sustained support for this project over an extended period of time. I appreciate Amy Sherman's and Alex Wolfe's careful guidance of the book production, Kimberly Laurel's skillful copyediting, and the beautiful cover design by Melissa Dias-Mandoly. For the maps that appear in this book, and other technical advice, many thanks to Ed Eastaugh, our department archaeology lab manager. Thanks to Ed, too, for reminding me that archaeologists have considerable experience in mapping change over time!

As a political anthropologist interested in how institutional processes work, and as a historical anthropologist interested in what shapes the documentary record, I have gradually come to understand that the considerable time I have spent in service roles at Western University—undoubtedly one reason I struggled to find the time and mental space to complete this book—has fundamentally shaped my understanding of the processes analyzed here. I don't know whether to thank or to blame colleagues who gave me the opportunity to lead our faculty union (for a three-year cycle), serve on the University Senate for several years, and take on leadership roles as department graduate program director (for three and a half years), department chair (for five years), and mostly recently, assistant dean. I know now that all of these experiences changed how I read archival documents, seeing in them traces of ongoing conversations and contestations, as fragments of *arguments* and not only evidence of events. This just confirms what I tell my undergraduate students in courses on the history of anthropology: we are all the product of the varied experiences we have had, many of which can shape our research in ways we may not immediately recognize.

I have been working in one way or another on this book's analysis for most (or all?) of Juliana, Marisol, and Alejandro's lives. Having shared research trips with them over two decades, now it's exciting to share more of my research results with them. This has taken so long that they have all grown from infants into potential readers of this work. They, and Fernando, make it all worthwhile.

Conjuring *the* State

Introduction

A 1929 photo of a public health encounter in the Ecuadorian highland Indigenous community Nisag, Alausí canton, Chimborazo province, helps introduce the themes of this book. The photo (see figure 1) was published in 1930 in the US journal *Public Health Reports*[1] and evokes the intersecting paths that came together in these encounters. Three men in suits can be seen. To the right is Dr. Carlos Miño, who led the first anti-plague campaign in the Alausí region in 1913, was the founding subdirector of the Quito branch office of public health from 1914 to 1925, and at the time of this photo was the national inspector general of public health. In the back is provincial public health delegate for Chimborazo, Dr. Alfonso Villagómez, who served for many years in this capacity before, in 1939, falling victim to a dramatic pneumonic plague outbreak in the provincial capital Riobamba that, within four days, killed him and all eleven nuns working at the provincial hospital. On the left is Dr. Clifford Eskey from the US Public Health Service, who in 1929–1930 co-led the American Commission with Pan American Sanitary Bureau physician Dr. John Long, working together with Ecuadorian public health experts to eliminate plague from the port city of Guayaquil. While the names of the individuals from Nisag are not provided, at the community level they had an equally situated identity as an autonomous community of "free Indians" (that is, not tied to *haciendas*, or large agricultural estates) with a history of resistance to and negotiation with municipal employees who, within a broader system of public works labor conscription,[2] had recruited them for anti-plague measures in the town of Alausí before their own village was infected. In the previous decade they had also actively resisted threats to their water supply and had been engaged in expanding their crop production by shrewdly taking advantage of agricultural development legislation that had been designed with the goal of benefiting much larger landowners.[3]

Public Health Reports, Vol. 45, No. 36, September 5, 1930

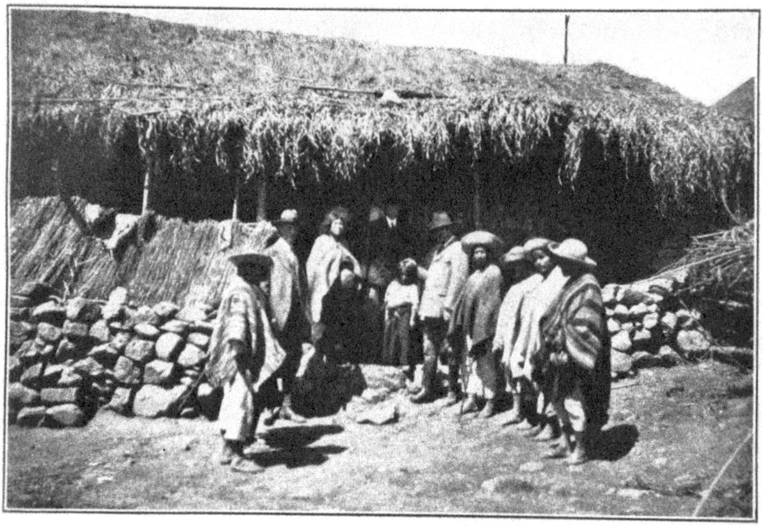

HUT AT NISAC IN WHICH A CASE OF PLAGUE WAS FOUND DECEMBER 15, 1929

Figure 1. Plague encounters in highland Ecuador: Nisag, Chimborazo, 1929.

In this book's discussion of public health encounters and state formation in Ecuador in the first decades of the twentieth century, the specificity of who came together in these encounters matters.[4] All participants whose paths intersected in these settings had prior histories that influenced their expectations and behavior, and their experience in one encounter could have an impact on how they approached the next one. While it is rarely possible to situate social actors with as much depth as one would like, the approach taken in this book attempts to treat them—working within limits set by the sources—as complexly motivated actors who drew on social knowledge and past experience in responding to emerging situations.[5] Of course, their intentional action often had unintended consequences, not least because others came to these encounters with their own interests and goals.

What kinds of people came together in encounters involving Ecuador's Servicio de Sanidad (Public Health Service)? What was the tone of their encounters? What helped or hindered the extension of public health programs? Importantly, archival documentation highlights that relevant encounters were not only between state actors and members of the public situated at two unproblematic poles. As the photo illustrates, they also involved encounters among institutional actors situated in particular ways in different government agencies. Sometimes actors in other government offices might push back against the Sanidad's entry into territory that they themselves previously occupied, revealing a dynamic of pressure and constraint as the institutional landscape was reshaped through these interactions and practices. Members of the Sanidad service had important encounters with the social actors embedded in the Beneficencia organization (social welfare; later, Asistencia Pública), municipal governments and councils, ministries and ministers, and universities as well as with a wide range of members of the Ecuadorian population affected by their projects. And sometimes those members of the public, too, were in shifting relations of tension and alliance with each other, giving the Sanidad a valuable opportunity to mediate. Together these encounters and processes helped conjure the state, making it seem real and functional to people, capable under some circumstances of intervening beneficially in their lives.

Approaches

The analysis presented here is located at the intersection of the concerns of historical anthropology and political anthropology. Historical anthropologists view the archive as encultured and situated; they are interested in what processes shaped the documentary record. Specifically in this book, a historical anthropology lens draws attention to how the archival record was formed through a proliferation of memos and orders between different state agencies, via communications among those differently positioned within a single agency, and in an interplay of petition and response between those targeted by state programs and those designing or delivering them. Using uncatalogued archives of correspondence is particularly rich for a project probing how the to-and-fro of everyday practices built up a matrix of resources for solving problems as it also built up and expressed (sometimes fraught) relationships.

From this perspective, the archive not only offers information about the past but also reveals elements of the ongoing shaping of institutional administrative processes.[6] It provides insights into how certain kinds of claims could be made and some forms of rule achieved, fundamental questions for political anthropology. Together, historical and political anthropology inform questions like: How did public health officials in different offices or regions coordinate their activities and communicate with each other? How did they manage relations with other actors—such as municipal governments, curative health care institutions, private physicians, and more—who crowded the landscape that they hoped to populate? How did information about health conditions get generated, collected, and compiled? How did the Sanidad develop a coherent institutional matrix (of personnel, channels of communication, forms of authority, and so on) with procedures that permitted it to generate, gather, and communicate information and then also to act on it? What kinds of complaints or requests could be lodged, using what mechanisms, and to whom were they directed? Focusing on questions of this kind, this book probes *how* things got done as much as it explores *what* got done.

The issues discussed in the chapters below were ones that asserted themselves insistently from an immersion in archival sources. They were chosen because of the amount of documentation generated about them, pointing to areas that were controversial or problematic or significant. From an anthropological perspective, the weight of these issues in the archive spoke of important problems for the public health service (and sometimes for the public itself). Of course, only a limited number of topics could be analyzed here. My 2012 book *Gender, State, and Medicine in Highland Ecuador* addresses a linked set of issues, specifically around gendered forms of social policy and state formation, that emerged from this same body of archival research, although it also led me along other archival paths. Readers will notice, too, that many of the processes foregrounded in the analysis of this book are not explicitly about confronting disease outbreaks, despite the fact that such events provided the rationale and motivation for the founding of the service. They include issues that perhaps would not catch the eye of a historian of public health but are deeply interesting to a political anthropologist. Completing this book in the midst of the COVID-19 pandemic highlighted quite viscerally the significance of questions about how things get done and how administrative action at different levels combines effectively to enable action, which may be an underappreciated dimension of past public health projects.

What does it mean to say that this is a study in the anthropology of the state, a historical institutional ethnography of the Ecuadorian Sanidad service? First, the *anthropology* in that phrase: the discipline's early cross-cultural and comparative focus revealed the immense variety of social forms and cultural practices among human societies, undermining notions that any particular way of organizing social life was normal. A basic premise of anthropology is thus that we should not assume that any social practice, social relation, or social institution is natural. Ultimately, this comparative perspective can prompt us to step back and ask how things came to be—including how they acquired the veneer of seeming natural, of just being part of the landscape. One of this book's starting points is that there is nothing obvious or inevitable about the state's ability to intervene in social relations, including when it comes to protecting health. Indeed, its capacity to do so in Ecuador evolved fairly quickly, and this book aims to understand what processes facilitated and deepened this capacity. Another founding approach in anthropology is ethnography—the detailed description of a society, rather than a comparison across societies—which emphasizes the insights that are gained by exploring social life through an examination of everyday practices, in the context of the relationships and environments in which they are embedded, and by endeavoring to see events and processes from the perspective of, and as they are experienced by, those directly involved.

How might we apply these general orientations to a historical anthropology of the *state*, given how far the study of a state agency is from the initial contexts in which anthropology's founding approaches were developed? We can start by exploring the perspectives and everyday practices of those involved in institutional processes, including those working for and those encountering the public health service. My analysis is based on a rich body of internal correspondence of the Sanidad, in which one can discern a great deal about the mundane practices of service employees, revealing how projects turn into policies and how policies are reshaped in the process of their implementation. While one might risk falling into triumphalism in foregrounding the perspective of public health physicians (who produced many of the documents used here), in fact the archival sources focus much more on the challenges they faced than on their successes, perhaps because these documents were generated in the midst of processes rather than retrospectively and were not intended for a public audience. The record shows that we cannot read off the consequences of state projects from their objectives, as the actions of the various social actors whose paths intersected in public health encounters produced something new that departed from what any of the actors might have intended. Importantly from the perspective of an anthropology of the state, the evidence from the sources documenting the everyday practices of state actors shows that changes to state procedures, policy, or law set conditions of possibility, enabled room for maneuver, and often yielded unexpected outcomes as social actors encountered each other under changing circumstances (which they further modified through their actions).

As one works through the archival record, it quickly becomes clear that infecto-contagious diseases were not the only problem the service was grappling with, although they were its reason for existing. How could service employees begin to confront diseases? How could they gather information that would allow them to interpret disease trends or, better yet, anticipate and prevent them? Who could they rely on to implement their disease eradication or prevention campaigns outside of the main cities—or even there? How could they secure sufficient resources to carry out their programs? And how might they predict who would be in a position to support their recommendations, particularly (but not only) in the era of acute political instability of the 1930s that saw frequent changes in the national government?

Are these simply problems of logistics? We might alternatively see them as challenges associated with developing an appropriate institutional structure to allow the public health service to act. How would our perspective change if we thought of Sanidad officials and employees not as cogs in the wheels of a well-oiled state machinery but as agents coming together and seeking to construct such a state, a project that might require both new institutional arrangements and the forging of particular images of the state? Historical sociologist Philip Abrams famously highlights two dimensions of state formation that he proposes are amenable to analysis. One is the state system, "a palpable nexus of practice and institutional structure centered in government"; at the same time, he insists that we should "recognize the cogency of the *idea* of the state," which should be studied along with the state system. Importantly, Abrams emphasizes the contingent features of both the state system and the state idea: the former is "*more or less* extensive, unified and dominant in any given society," while the latter is "projected, purveyed and *variously believed* in different societies at different times."[7] Abrams's doctoral students Philip Corrigan and Derek Sayer demonstrate the new research questions and insights that this kind of analysis could generate in their now-classic study *The Great Arch: English State Formation as Cultural Revolution*.[8] Reading the Ecuadorian material through the lens of Abrams's distinction suggests a further question: How might the state system and state idea relate to each other? How did changes to the state idea and state system build on each other iteratively in a process of mutual reshaping? If a particular idea of the state was communicated by certain state actors, how could it be used to press other officials to live up to it? Might this extend arenas for state action, partly by means of people appealing to proliferating numbers of differently positioned personnel as the state system was built up across the national territory?[9] While the ongoing shaping of a state idea plays an important role in the story that follows, there is perhaps even more attention to the laborious assembling of a state system that would permit action, something that too often is assumed rather than analyzed in studies of state processes.

Abrams also argues that the state is, at the end of the day, "first and foremost an exercise in legitimation. . . . The state is not the reality which stands behind the mask of political practice. It is itself the mask, which prevents our seeing political practice as it is."[10] Analyses of contested hegemony by historians and anthropologists of Latin America have broadly influenced my thinking about processes that contribute to that legitimation. Historian Gilbert Joseph and anthropologist Daniel Nugent bring together groundbreaking contributions to this literature in their 1994 volume *Everyday Forms of State Formation*.[11] The authors engage with the work of historical sociologists Abrams, Sayer, and Corrigan in rethinking domination and resistance in Mexico. They also extend the foundational analysis of Antonio Gramsci (as do Corrigan and Sayer), emphasizing especially that hegemonic processes are partial and ongoing and more often projects than stable achievements. Influential work followed, further complicating our understanding of hegemony and resistance and foregrounding complex dynamics of reciprocity and repression, resistance and accommodation, and evasion and confrontation in the historical formation of Latin American nations. Exemplary work on the interplay of national projects and alternative peasant nationalisms was contributed by historians Florencia Mallon on Mexico and Peru and Greg Grandin on Guatemala.[12] For Ecuador, also advancing a broadly Gramscian analysis, historian Valeria Coronel emphasizes the importance of coalitions and social alliances in shaping the political field in the first half of the twentieth century.[13] In a recent suggestive analysis, Pablo Ospina Peralta furthers the application of Gramsci to Ecuadorian state processes by viewing the middle decades of the twentieth century through the lens of Gramsci's concept of *trasformismo*, especially highlighting the fragile compromises and shifting negotiations underlying Ecuador's political history.[14] For the Andes more broadly, the essays collected in *State Theory and Andean Politics* by anthropologists Christopher Krupa and David Nugent deepen our understanding of contested hegemony from what they call an "off-centered" perspective.[15] Influenced by this body of work, I have been particularly interested in exploring the micropolitical processes through which those advancing hegemonic projects seek to dominate some opposing groups and, perhaps more importantly, to lead other allied groups.[16] To do so may involve modifying governing projects to include, if only partially, the aspirations of a variety of groups, a point that historian Paulo Drinot also makes effectively in his study of race, nation, and labor in Peru.[17] In the kinds of encounters through which these processes were actualized, those projects themselves might be extended and reshaped. Through their actions in the matrix of a developing state system, Ecuadorian public health officials also contributed to establishing a notion of the state as separate from society and standing above it, demonstrating its ability to intervene when they helped people address some of the everyday dilemmas they faced. Many scholars have referred to these as state effects.

In this analysis, I am also inspired by the work of non–Latin Americanist scholars who have challenged us to consider the everyday practices and social and cultural effects of state formation in ways that help us see the state as an ethnographic space. Anthropologists' emphasis on everyday practices has been applied to institutional contexts by sociologist Dorothy Smith through her institutional ethnography method of inquiry.[18] Smith writes of the social quite explicitly as the coordination of people's doings. This raises the key question of what it meant, in early twentieth-century Ecuador, for public health leaders to coordinate their actions sufficiently to function as an institution. Smith also reminds us of the central role of texts—by which she means information in a format that enables replication and storage—in coordinating people's doings over time and across distances, simultaneously present in their everyday worlds and connecting them to translocal social relations. This is especially important for the study of institutions since, as Smith would say, in institutional settings people are actively producing the general out of the particular. We can see this in the burgeoning statistical production of Sanidad officials who sought to bring together and align disparate data to decipher population trends. Smith also emphasizes how distinctive institutional modes of generalizing coordination are brought into being in people's doings at particular sites and times. This aligns well with how historical anthropologists' queries about the shaping of the documentary record intersect with political anthropologists' attention to how things get done.

Political geographer Joe Painter also highlights how an analysis of everyday or prosaic practices can enhance our understanding of state formation.[19] Painter argues that such an approach helps to break down assumptions of separate spheres—that the state occupies a distinct and identifiable segment of the social whole that then interacts with other distinct social spheres—thus disrupting the binary logic of state/non-state formulations. Understanding states through prosaic practices undermines reification, revealing their heterogeneous, constructed, porous, uneven, processual, and relational character and highlighting the actual practices through which social relations of stateness are reproduced. For instance, he points out that passing legislation has few immediate effects in itself. "Rather, its effects are produced in practice through the myriad mundane actions of officials, clerks, police officers, inspectors, teachers, social workers, doctors, and so on. In addition, the act of passing legislation in the first place also depends on the prosaic practices and small decisions of parliamentary drafters, elected politicians, civil servants and all those who influence them, including journalists, electors, letter writers, campaigning organizations, lobbyists, academics and others. . . . Thus the outcome of state actions is always uncertain and fallible."[20] Painter further argues that "the production of state effects . . . depends not only on myriad mundane and prosaic practices, but also on these practices successfully combining in the particular time-space configuration that will enable" administrative action.[21] This key point is compatible with Smith's attention to the processes involved in the combining or coordinating of activities. Interestingly, Painter seems to identify Abrams's contribution primarily in terms of his highlighting of the state idea,[22] despite how Abrams's emphasis on the state system points to the development of a matrix of offices and personnel, and the practices in which they engage, consistent with Painter's concerns.

Painter and Abrams turn the autonomy and unity of the state into a research question rather than treating it as a natural occurrence; similarly, political scientist Timothy Mitchell proposes that the seeming autonomy of the state and its separation from society is a powerful state effect that itself should be subject to analysis in historically specific contexts.[23] In probing how the state might come to seem that way, Painter phrases it this way: the state in whose name officials function is "a symbolic resource on which they draw to produce their effects."[24] Still, Painter comments that these effects themselves, what he calls *stateness*, "is not an illusion, but is actualized in countless mundane social and material practices within and outside the institutions conventionally referred to as the state apparatus."[25] It is not only the state that is reified in this process, as it seems to become separate from society—the other abstraction produced simultaneously is society. How this occurred in a particular time and place—Ecuador in the early twentieth century—is at the heart of this book, pursued through a study that also provides new historical information about processes inherently interesting in their own right, such as bubonic plague outbreaks in specific moments and regional spaces in Ecuador. In applying these suggestive concepts to the study of Ecuadorian state formation, I agree with Painter that this is not an illusion. In fact, I am interested in understanding what we might call "real people doing real things with real consequences"—a project in which an ethnographically inspired approach focuses attention on the mundane social and material practices that Painter and Smith highlight.

Finally, the emphasis on public health draws our attention to relations of care in ways that may be more generally relevant for an understanding of state processes. In *Fevers, Feuds, and Diamonds*, Paul Farmer distinguishes between containment and care in disease eradication programs.[26] He highlights this contrast in his discussion of Ebola in West Africa, where *containment* of spread was emphasized and clinical treatment or *care* was limited, even though supportive care such as rehydration would have been generally viable even where the greater technology needed for critical care might have been unavailable. For Ebola, containment and care were often treated as competing tasks rather than complementary ones—for instance, when control of spread led to a no-touch policy that eliminated basic supportive care and left patients to rehydrate themselves, something that they were often too weak to manage.[27] This general framework contrasting control or containment and care is extended here from the discussion of approaches to a single disease to a broader set of questions about how the public health agency in Ecuador positioned itself and went about its evolving responsibilities. In Ecuador the Sanidad worked on disease prevention and eradication in uneasy tension with the agency who managed healthcare institutions (Beneficencia), whose mandate was more directly *care* in the sense of treatment. Nonetheless, the analysis of Ecuadorian processes demonstrates the importance for the Sanidad to pursue a broader form of care in order to advance containment or control of disease.[28] Most significantly, this was captured in Sanidad officials' ability to help resolve difficulties and thus to position themselves and the agency as mediator or facilitator within a dynamic matrix of social actors.

In some ways I began this book's analysis in my 2012 study *Gender, State, and Medicine in Highland Ecuador.* There I examined several health-related arenas in which women became either objects or agents of state formation and gendered social policy. The former included child health and welfare as well as prostitution regulation and venereal disease control programs. The latter included professional midwives who worked for the public health service in its maternal-infant health programs as well as nurses who worked for state hospitals. Midwives and nurses also received their training in state institutions, and as such they were themselves the objects or products of gendered social policy initiatives. Throughout, I was interested in how state agents' social backgrounds and private lives might influence their actions within public health and medical institutions, which helps collapse the seeming separation between state and society. I also emphasized the multiplicity of social positions and varied intentions that might be encompassed in a state institution, undermining the notion that the state has a single and unproblematic set of interests and intentions. Here, I extend my analysis to include an exploration of how a notion of the state as separate from society—a reification of the state—was constructed in Ecuador, through the lens of an examination of one state agency. The Sanidad lends itself particularly well to such an analysis as its physician leaders were preoccupied with developing a more robust institutional structure that would allow them to act. They also seemed to be acutely aware of the importance of the

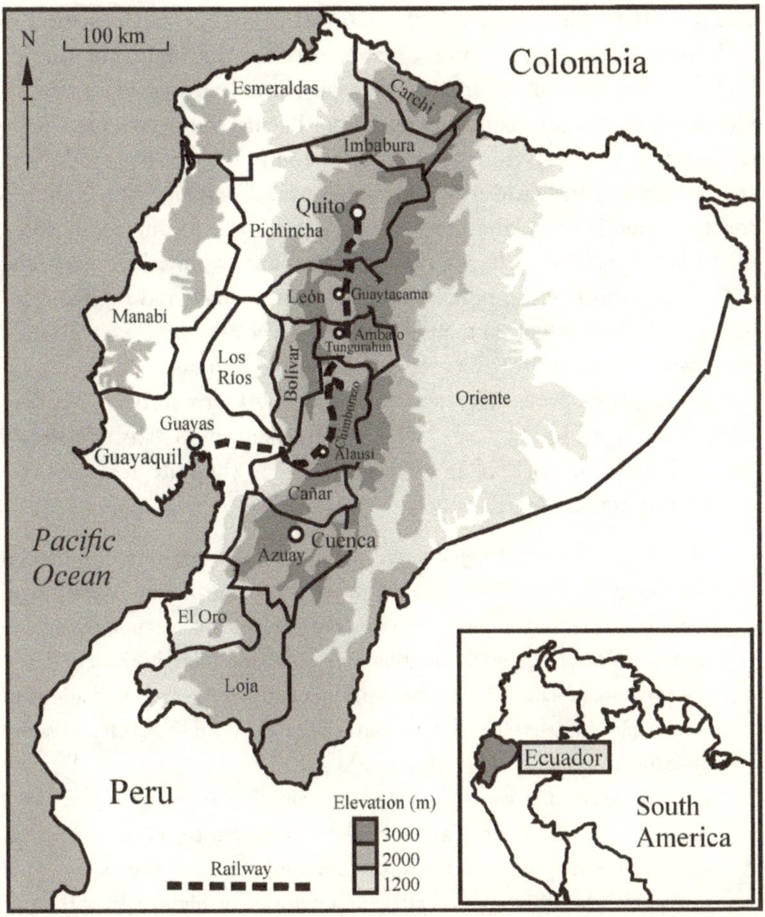

Map 1. Ecuador in 1920. This map presents the names and shapes of provinces as of 1920, with the exclusion of the eastern portion of the Amazonian territory that was lost to Peru in 1941 and the Galápagos Islands (neither of which figure into the book's narrative). ***Credit:*** **Edward Eastaugh.**

image of the state produced through their actions and were concerned with who could speak for or represent the state.[29]

Region, Health, and Disease in Ecuador

As problems that involve human beings and other biological organisms, diseases and medical conditions emerge in specific kinds of climates, landscapes, and regional spaces. Crossed by the equator and divided by the Andean cordillera running north–south, Ecuador has significant geographic and climatic diversity in a relatively small territory. In the center of the country, the double chain of the Andes divides the Ecuadorian mainland into three distinct regions: the highlands (*sierra*), including two rows of mountain peaks with cross-cutting ridges that divide the inter-Andean zone into numerous basins; the coastal plain (*costa* or *litoral*) to the west, from the Pacific Ocean to the western foothills of the Andes; and the eastern Amazonian lowlands (*oriente*). The country's fourth region is the Galapagos archipelago off the Pacific coast, about 600 kilometers west of the mainland. In the early twentieth century (and still today), most of the population lived in the coast and highland regions, and hence attention to public health in the decades covered by this book was almost entirely focused on these two regions.

In his 1892 geography text on Ecuador, German-born Teodoro Wolf, contracted by the Ecuadorian government in 1870 as a professor for the Polytechnic School and later also named the state geologist, describes the highlands this way:

> The great longitudinal valley between the eastern and western cordilleras is not continuous but rather divided into extensive basins by transverse ridges that cross over and connect the two cordilleras at various points and rise up to considerable heights over the basins. . . . The central region of Ecuador presents in nature a physical appearance that is highly varied and with surprising contrasts, as occurs in countries of an Alpine character. Pleasant plateaus, irrigated with gentle streams and shaded by orange and myrtle trees, are crossed by valleys and steep canyons, in whose depths rush noisy torrents, and the flanks of the cordilleras rise from the cheerful plateaus with their wheat and corn fields, up to the inhospitable wastelands of the *páramos* [high-altitude grasslands] and finally to the high peaks of the volcanoes, crowned with perpetual snow.

The coastal plain, he emphasizes, was very different:

> This zone, which in the south . . . is two or three leagues wide, from the latitude of Guayaquil broadens to thirty leagues or more. Not all of the region is flat, although there exist extensive plains especially in the fluvial system of the Guayas River and the lower stretches of other large rivers; rather, the landscape is generally mountainous . . . the hills forming undulating landscapes. What most defines this region is the multitude of navigable rivers, which in many areas of dense vegetation are the only routes of communication and transport. The grand and wild vistas of the high altitudes are lacking, predominating instead the pleasant landscapes of tropical vegetation.[30]

Writing a decade later, US diplomat Thomas Dawson adds that "the Ecuador coast is one of the most fertile and lovely regions on the earth. It already furnishes a considerable proportion of those tropical products of which the great nations of the temperate zone demand more every year. . . . Its green shores refresh the eyes of the north-bound traveler tired of the dreary desert that stretches from Valparaiso to the Gulf of Guayaquil; it possesses the best harbor on the Pacific south of Panama and one of the few in all South America which is not mountain-locked." With his interest in South America's commercial prospects, Dawson notes that "between the Cordillera and the sea there is room for untold millions of cacao and coffee trees."[31]

Settlement patterns and social relations evolved differently in the regional spaces of the highlands and the coast. The highlands had settled Indigenous agricultural populations that were in the process of being incorporated into the expanding Inca Empire in the decades before the arrival of the Spaniards. Building on these earlier patterns of relatively dense Indigenous occupation, in the colonial period the highlands continued to be home to greater population densities and economic activity, since access to Indigenous labor underlay the regional colonial economy, based on textile production and agriculture to supply internal colonial circuits. Following independence, the highland economy contracted with the dismantling of the colonial circuits of trade and transition to new forms of international integration. Characteristic images of the highlands in the nineteenth century would include the large Indigenous peasant population living in villages abutting large estates or as a dependent population tied to those estates via debt peonage (*concertaje*) and tenancy (*huasipungaje*). Although there were aristocratic creole[32] families with a long tradition of owning large properties, the largest landowner in the highlands in the nineteenth century was the Catholic Church, whose rural estates provisioned its urban institutions. Indeed, the Church also had a strong influence on urban society in the highlands, with its domination over education and its numerous churches and convents.[33] Agriculture in the highlands was oriented toward regional markets rather than export, land use was extensive, and incipient industry (such as textile production and leather manufacturing) was largely linked to agriculture. Transport and travel were costly and slow. As a result, it was only after the inauguration of the railway between Guayaquil and Quito in 1908 that the transport of heavy equipment and construction materials enabled the modernization of the colonial-era city of Quito in the north-central highlands.

The coastal economy and society were different in significant ways. In the rural areas, export-oriented cacao (cocoa) plantations expanded rapidly in the second half of the nineteenth century, becoming an important engine of economic growth for independent Ecuador. The network of waterways crossing the tropical plain meant that little fixed infrastructure was necessary. The fact that the ocean tides moved up the Guayas River well inland meant that the flow of the river changed direction with the tides, enabling transport by rafts even before steam-powered paddlewheels began to transport goods and travelers in the 1860s. Other tropical export goods were also produced on the coast, such as tagua (vegetable ivory or ivory nut) and rubber. The growth of Guayaquil port and the city itself was fed by the active trade in these products, and the city hosted many commercial import-export establishments that made available a wide range of foreign goods to local elites, who had considerable disposable incomes from the export economy. The region also attracted migrants from other areas, both for urban economic opportunities in Guayaquil and for the expansion of agro-export production in the countryside of the coastal provinces. An argument could be made that coastal society—with the lesser weight of Catholic influence, the greater mobility of people, and sustained relations with other regions through import, export, and travel—was "naturally" more liberal than the highlands. And indeed, the liberal period took the form of the rise of coastal interests over highland ones, with attacks on the Catholic Church and on the privileges of traditional highland elites, described further below.

Health conditions also differed across these regions. The humid coastal plain—distinctive from the dry coastal region farther south in Peru, as Dawson emphasizes—also contrasted significantly with the Andean region with its drier and cooler environment. As the main entry point for goods and people due to its excellent harbor, the reputation of the tropical port of Guayaquil as the "pesthole of the Pacific" in the early twentieth century had more than local significance.[34] As construction work progressed on the Panama Canal (which would be inaugurated in 1914), health conditions all along the western coast of South America came under increasing international scrutiny.

In 1903, physician Hugh S. Cumming of the US Public Health and Marine-Hospital Service (PHMHS)—who would go on to be appointed both surgeon general of the United States and director of the Pan American Sanitary Bureau in 1920, leading the latter organization for twenty-seven years[35]—reported on some of the dangers for Panama and the United States posed by commercial traffic along the west coast of South and Central America. He highlighted particularly the weekly arrivals in Panama of the vessels of the Pacific Steam Navigation and South American Steamship companies that had stopped at ports in Chile, Peru, Ecuador, and Colombia. In relation to the recent arrival of plague on the west coast of the Americas, he pointed out that along the whole west coast from San Diego down to Chile there was no quarantine station and, given the "vast trade already centering" in 1903 at Panama, he recommended appointing a sanitary inspector of the PHMHS to operate in the Canal Zone.[36] The next year a US consular official in Guayaquil elaborates:

> The certainty of completion of the isthmian canal gives to Guayaquil a position, from a sanitary standpoint, not possessed a few years ago. She becomes an important factor in all that concerns the sanitation of the Canal Zone and one which must be dealt with intelligently in order to obtain the desired results on the Isthmus. Her commercial importance, which brings her in frequent communication with the Isthmus, only 700 miles distant, is already great and with the opening of the canal will rank her of first importance among the cities on the Pacific side of South America, among which she now ranks third after Valparaíso and Callao.[37]

Indeed, ports were key points of entry and control when it came to diseases. In the mid- and late nineteenth century, international sanitary agreements had the primary goal of ensuring reliable exchange of information specifically to protect ports. While terrestrial *cordons sanitaires* (restrictions on movement to prevent the spread of disease) could work for some diseases, ports were more vulnerable to pathogens coming from distant locations. Expansion in international commerce and the increased speed and shortened distances involved in transportation in the nineteenth century were important factors in the spread of diseases, stimulating preventive measures through control of trade and travel. International agreements involved both quarantine provisions and compulsory notification of outbreaks of specific diseases: cholera, yellow fever, smallpox, and bubonic plague. Hence, too, the growing importance of marine health officers, whose role was to inspect ships and passengers and issue bills of health for ships embarking for ports in specific countries.

Massive fires affected Guayaquil at the turn of the nineteenth century, which had implications for health. In October 1896 a fire gutted ninety-two city blocks and, following the previous year's Liberal Revolution, led the constituent assembly meeting in Guayaquil to regularize rule to decamp and move to Quito. Another city-wide fire in July 1902 destroyed twenty-six city blocks.[38] By 1904 the result was significant:

> Guayaquil of today is not the same as Guayaquil of ten years ago. Successive great fires have visited the city and changed its appearance. Contrasting the unburned district with the new or rebuilt section, it cannot be denied that the visitation of fire has done much to improve this city in every way. Thus the city presents the appearance of two distinct towns in

> one. The new or rebuilt section with broad, raised streets, for the most part well paved and partially drained; the houses large, well built, and with excellent accommodations for light and ventilation, and supplied with water-closets and baths. The old part, with crooked, narrow, and ill-paved streets, is, for the greater part, without sewers. The houses are poorly ventilated and overcrowded and offer every facility for the propagation of disease. In these there is almost a total absence of modern water-closets. Again there is another part of Guayaquil which is altogether unhealthy, insanitary, and filthy. This third section is on the outskirts of the city. The streets are low, without any attempt at sewage, and with many stagnant pools. The houses are poorly built, unsanitary, and in great part overcrowded and dirty. The roofs are covered with cadi, a kind of palm which becomes the abiding place of various insects. The lots are all below the street level.[39]

The post-fire renovation of architecture among Guayaquil's wealthier inhabitants was undoubtedly helpful in some ways, but the fact that many poor residents were made homeless by fire encouraged the spread of other diseases in the subsequent rainy seasons. In addition, the influx of nonimmune construction workers from other regions to rebuild the city may well have fueled the yellow fever epidemics.[40]

The 1908 arrival of bubonic plague in Guayaquil, discussed in the next chapter, was the direct catalyst for the establishment that year of Ecuador's Servicio de Sanidad. As the director general of Sanidad made explicit to the Fifth International Sanitary Convention of the American Republics three years later in Chile: "The arrival of plague in Guayaquil in 1908 marked a new era in public health institutions" in Ecuador. He also explained the decision to locate the service in Guayaquil: "The circumstance that the port of Guayaquil is the commercial metropolis of the republic, whose population is continually renewed by foreigners and migrants from the country's interior who are not immune to yellow fever, and above all the alarm created by the ravages caused by the plague in this port, determined the creation of the Servicio de Sanidad Pública whose headquarters resides in Guayaquil."[41] Plague joined yellow fever in Guayaquil as two diseases that were of obligatory disclosure under international sanitary agreements. A third such disease, smallpox, was eradicated in the city of Guayaquil in 1909 (although it continued to persist in several other Ecuadorian locations for some time).[42] Among these diseases, yellow fever was eliminated in 1919, but plague proved to be challenging as chapter 1 shows.

In his 1911 address to the Fifth International Sanitary Convention, Ecuador's director general of Sanidad highlighted the very different situation of the highlands and the coast when it came to health threats:

> In Ecuador there is a marked difference in demographic statistics in the cities located in the inter-Andean region [*meseta*] and those of the coastal cities. This difference favors considerably the former, when it comes to morbidity and mortality, which is easily explainable by the special nature of the high-altitude climate, unsuitable for the propagation of yellow fever, because there the *stegomya* does not exist; less apt to the evolution of malaria, because the radius of the *anopheles* is limited to certain valleys; and because the highland climate is more favorable to combat successfully the ravages of tuberculosis. In the interior of the republic one lives under the healthy influence of a climate of perpetual springtime; the coast suffers instead the rude heat of the tropical environment.[43]

He went on to highlight how this was represented by the different health conditions in the highland capital city Quito and the port city Guayaquil (undoubtedly it was only in these two cities that sufficient data would have been available to allow him to estimate incidence of disease). He explained that the general rate of mortality in the city of Quito (with an estimated population at the time of eighty thousand) was 2.37 per thousand, with the most important causes of death being bronchitis, pneumonia, and dysentery. The weight of infecto-contagious diseases in general mortality was low: 0.40 percent of deaths were caused by tuberculosis, 0.03 percent by typhoid fever, 0.02 percent by smallpox, and 0.01 percent by malaria. In contrast, in Guayaquil in 1910 the similarly sized population of some eighty-two thousand residents faced a mortality rate of 41.18 per thousand. The most significant causes of mortality were tuberculosis at 13.79 percent of the total mortality, malaria at 9.78 percent, plague at 8.58 percent, and yellow fever at 4.61 percent. The director pointed out that Guayaquil received large numbers of patients from elsewhere in its medical establishments, which contributed to these alarming figures.[44] Still, the contrast between regions is stark.

Some issues examined in this book are of national scope, with a special emphasis on how the highland and coastal regions were connected via the circulation of personnel, experiences, resources, and even diseases (the Amazon region was largely overlooked in public health programs for most of the period covered in this book). However, in the chapters that follow I focus especially on the highlands for others. Given the contrasts in health conditions outlined above, this would be a very different book—undoubtedly concentrating much more on tropical diseases—if it emphasized primarily the coast. The highland focus helps to clarify the many other issues faced by the Sanidad that are relevant to this book's political anthropology questions, which might have been obscured by the weight of infecto-contagious diseases on the coast.[45] My 2012 book

Gender, State, and Medicine in Highland Ecuador examines some of the highlands' tenacious health problems, for instance those contributing to infant mortality and those associated with venereal diseases, in the context of evolving relations between state programs and women's experience and actions. Here I extend that analysis into other areas, including the micropolitics underlying the establishment and extension over space of public health programs, which are explored through the detailed record left of the public health service's everyday practices.

Political Change in Ecuador

Because the story of public health is centrally the story of a state agency, changes in government and general political orientation could have profound effects on how public health was conceptualized, funded, and operationalized. Public health as a national endeavor in Ecuador was a creation of the liberal period in 1895–1925. An important precursor of state modernization in other areas, however, was the paradoxical conservative president Gabriel García Moreno, who came to power after the near dissolution of the national territory in 1859 (when four juntas claimed to govern the country from different regional spaces) and dominated national politics from 1860 until his assassination in 1875. His was a new kind of conservatism inspired by his observations in exile of the aftereffects of the 1848 revolutions in Europe and his favorable impressions of the autocratic regime of Napoleon III.[46] He set out to modernize Ecuador through infrastructure programs, extension of primary education, and reform of advanced education with the contracting of European religious orders and the establishment of the Polytechnic School in Quito. He strengthened the central state—for instance, mobilizing Indigenous conscript labor in his road-building program (in the wake of the 1857 abolition of Indigenous tribute), which helped integrate regions while it also undermined highland landowners' control over Indigenous laborers. This process also bolstered municipal mechanisms to manage labor recruitment while other elements of municipal autonomy (such as around the control of budgeting) were weakened in this period. In addition, he dismantled Ecuador's previous tripartite structure of large districts in favor of expanding the number of provinces, which had the effect of multiplying the number of government officials across those administrative units. It was precisely in this period when some other Latin American countries were experimenting with liberal social and political reforms such as the separation of church and state, which occurred alongside forms of economic liberalization associated with export-led development that expanded in the 1870s. Ecuador instead was undergoing an experiment in tying the state closer to the Catholic Church under García Moreno, who dedicated the country to the sacred heart of Jesus and worked to establish an "empire of morality,"[47] at the same time as he promoted other reforms to infrastructure, education, and administrative processes that had a more modernizing bent. This formed part of the backdrop against which early twentieth century initiatives were undertaken.

In the highlands, nonetheless, it is important to note that prior to the 1895 Liberal Revolution many tasks that we would associate with governing processes continued to be privatized in the hands of either the Catholic Church or highland landowners. For instance, the Church controlled vital statistics information in its parish registries, and only with the 1900 Law of Civil Registry did it become obligatory to register births, deaths, and marriages with a state agency. Such information was relevant for the transmission of property as well as fundamentally important for the state's incipient knowledge of the health (and even the size) of the population. Highland landowners, in turn, controlled many aspects of peasant life on their large estates, from economic activities to the regulation of personal lives (including permission to marry). Liberal governments' emphasis on the rights of labor can be seen as in part due to their conviction that Indigenous labor was tied up unproductively in highland estates and that it could be employed more beneficially to advance export production on the coast.[48] Early liberal moves to loosen landowner control over labor included the requirement to register labor contracts with government officials, although the heritability of debt by means of which estate owners tied generations of peasants to their estates was not abolished until 1918. The strengthening of notions of state jurisdiction over public health in the early twentieth century was thus occurring alongside other significant changes such as the separation of church and state and the transformation of labor regimes.

The 1895 Liberal Revolution brought to power coastal agro-export and commercial elites who generally sought to modernize and open up the economy. Different emphases and alliances characterized the governments of the leaders who dominated the two decades after the Liberal Revolution: Eloy Alfaro, president in 1895–1901 and 1906–1911; and Leonidas Plaza, president in 1901–1905 and 1912–1916. Nonetheless, their governments largely shared an emphasis on secularization and modernization. At the same time, the decade of the 1910s saw substantial financial problems in Ecuador that interfered with public health programs and many other projects. In 1913 and 1914, the national government was engaged in fighting a civil war in the central and northern coastal provinces of Manabí and Esmeraldas. Then, with the advent of the First World War in 1914, government revenues plummeted with the reduction in Ecuadorian cacao exports, the paralysis of the international trade in tagua (or ivory nut) centered in Hamburg, Germany, and the diversion of British merchant vessels for the war effort. Soon after the war ended, the expansion of crop diseases in the coastal cacao plantations was another blow, further undermining exports. These economic factors in part underlay government indebtedness to private banks in Guayaquil and what was perceived as the increasing control of this "*bancocracia*" over government policies. Labor conflicts were another expression of the economic situation—and a massacre of striking workers in Guayaquil in 1922 powerfully symbolized the displacement of the more radical aspects of the liberal project by repression and corruption.

In 1925 another fundamental political shift came with the Revolución Juliana, or July Revolution, when a nationalist cohort of midranking military officers joined with middle-class professionals to overthrow the liberals in a bloodless coup. In terms of health issues, the coup elevated physician Isidro Ayora—the first Ecuadorian doctor to undertake specialist training in obstetrics—to the newly established position of minister of social welfare and then to the national presidency from 1926 to 1931. The Juliana governments between 1925 and 1931 engaged in an energetic process of reform, establishing Ecuador's Central Bank, nationalizing the Guayaquil-Quito railway, and passing social legislation that, for instance, regulated working conditions and institutionalized female suffrage (the latter, a first in Latin America). Their administrative reforms involved coordination and harmonizing of state institutions, including a reorganization of the Sanidad service that moved its main office from Guayaquil to Quito and created provincial delegations to extend public health programs beyond Ecuador's main cities. For plague in particular this led to the arrival of the American Commission and increased cooperation with Peruvian authorities in 1929–1930. The sanitation of Guayaquil by the British firm White,[49] which took longer than anticipated due to the financial problems that began in the mid-1910s, was also concluded in this period. Altogether, these reforms produced a more active, interventionist state, one effect of which was the considerable expansion of state employment, especially in Quito.[50] I agree with historian Coronel that this period is less interesting in terms of traditional Ecuadorian historiographic questions about whether it constituted a transfer of power from coastal to highland elites and more important for the new mechanisms that were established in processes of governance that, in her case in rural areas, "permitted peasant communities and workers to access new legal and political mechanisms to process their conflicts."[51] I argue that for urban areas in particular, the expanding matrix of officials who facilitated the resolution of conflicts included those working for the Sanidad service.

Coronel has also generally argued that the post-Juliana years saw a shift in Ecuadorian political life from a period when the main axis of political conflict was between liberals and conservatives to one where that axis involved the left (increasingly strengthened by alliances with peasants and workers) and conservatives.[52] From a different angle, Ospina Peralta also offers fascinating insight into how the charged field of force involving a broadly liberal-affiliated military institution and conservative politicians shaped political relations and the atmosphere of instability in the 1930s.[53] This instability was particularly notable in that decade as the country experienced a generalized economic crisis that was matched by an extraordinary degree of political volatility: there were fifteen men who passed through the presidential offices in rapid succession in that decade alone. The economic difficulties that were provoked in part by the trade disruptions during the First World War were deepened first with the spread of crop diseases in coastal cacao plantations, then with the Great Depression. Although this was a "bust" period between Ecuador's earlier boom of cacao and a later agro-export boom of banana production that took off in the late 1940s, scholars have recognized a diverse set of experiences of this period.[54] In a context where global trade was reduced due to the Depression, there were efforts to expand industrial production of textiles and other consumer goods. There was also considerable migration to urban areas such as Quito. The decade was marked, too, by the emergence of populism, based on the social transformations associated with urban growth, economic change, and diversification. Meanwhile, new forms of labor organizing were percolating that connected urban workers and rural peasants. At the scale of the national political system, in a way relative political stability emerged at the end of the decade under Carlos Arroyo del Río whose presidency lasted four years from 1940 to 1944, but the loss of half of Ecuador's territory (in the Amazon region) to Peru in a 1941 war was one of the catalysts for another political revolution. The Revolución Gloriosa of 1944 brought populist José María Velasco Ibarra back to the presidency for the second of his five terms. In 1948, the election of Galo Plaza Lasso (president from 1948 to 1952), a modernizing landowner who was the son of former liberal president Plaza, initiated an extended phase of political stability, based in part on the consolidation of the banana boom in the 1950s.

International factors and context played a role in many of the processes discussed in this book. As a signatory to multilateral sanitary conventions, Ecuador had to follow international regulations to disclose incidents of certain diseases. Some diseases themselves came from abroad. Meetings with international colleagues were important venues for sharing experiences, and advanced training in foreign institutions was also increasingly common among Ecuadorian physicians. In some cases, foreign researchers and physicians participated directly in Ecuadorian eradication campaigns, such as the 1929 American Commission that undertook anti-plague work alongside Ecuadorian public health officials. All of these international factors can be clearly seen in Ecuador's encounter with plague, explored in the next chapter, but even there the international processes did not determine what occurred in Ecuador. Indeed, as a biological organism developing in local environments, the disease ecology of plague was itself different in Ecuador than elsewhere. Moreover, plague was combatted by Ecuadorians, in Ecuadorian ways, and through Ecuadorian interactions and negotiations.

In thinking about the relative influence of international actors, it is worth noting that there was not a significant weight of foreign investment in Ecuador at the time. As historian Ronn Pineo points out, Ecuador's most important export product, cacao, relied on the natural conditions on the coast and needed little processing prior to shipping, with the result that the expansion of plantations was within the means of the emerging coastal elite rather than dependent on large infusions of foreign capital.[55] Indeed, the principal US enterprise in Ecuador in the first two decades of the twentieth century was not an export-producing venture at all: it was the private US company Guayaquil and Quito Railway, which completed construction of the railroad to Quito in 1908. The railway project was subject to an extraordinary level of internal controversy, given its cost and the significant irregularities in both its construction and its operation.[56] The US State Department did not remain neutral in the resulting conflicts: in 1912, for instance, the US government sent a warship to Ecuadorian waters, with authorization to land troops if necessary to protect US interests. Attempts to resolve ongoing disputes between the company and the Ecuadorian government through international arbitration failed, and the US government continued to exert pressure on Ecuador, including carrying through on its threats to have the War Trade Board suspend imports of Ecuadorian cacao to the US in 1918, in a context in which the Ecuadorian export economy had already been damaged by the indirect effects of the war in Europe.[57] Sometimes the railway conflict impacted public health directly: for instance, in 1915 when the Ecuadorian government set aside 40 percent of import duties for the sanitation of Guayaquil, the US government lodged a formal protest against the use of customs revenues for anything other than payment of overdue (but bitterly disputed) interest on the railway bonds.[58] By 1923 the British consul in Quito reported to the Foreign Office in London that "the American nation is in no way popular with the Ecuadorians, who constantly fear that the United States will on one pretext or another, preferably the railway, intervene and treat this country as it has done with Nicaragua and other unfortunate Central American states who have fallen under its Monroe doctrine."[59] Finally in 1925, the Ecuadorian government purchased the majority share in the railway when the company claimed that it could not repair damage done to the line by landslides during the rainy season (during an El Niño year, typically characterized by heavy rainfall, flooding, and landslides). The government proceeded to repair the line at a much lower cost, and much more quickly, than the company had said was possible.

Unlike in Africa and South Asia, or even some parts of the Caribbean, in Ecuador (as in many Latin American countries), leading public health actors were not colonizers but conationals, although they might differ in class, ethnic, or sometimes gendered ways from the targets of their programs. In 1906, President Alfaro invited US technical assistance in dealing with the yellow fever situation in Guayaquil. It was agreed that the governor of the Canal Zone and sanitary officer Colonel William C. Gorgas would confer with the authorities of Guayaquil on sanitary reform. However, the idea was so unpopular when it became known that the matter was dropped.[60] In 1913, the Rockefeller Foundation's International Health Commission was launched with hookworm campaigns in Central America and the Caribbean.[61] The Foundation focused its energies initially on campaigns against specific diseases, such as hookworm, yellow fever, and malaria, and increasingly also invested in medical education through support for institutions in other countries and scholarships for medical practitioners from such countries to study in North America. While there was Rockefeller involvement in the eradication of yellow fever in Guayaquil in 1919, it was undertaken under the guise of a study rather than an eradication campaign[62] given local sensibilities around US policies toward Ecuador in recent years, as outlined above. Historian Steven Palmer argues that early Rockefeller projects in the Caribbean were less top-down and more open to local engagements and negotiations than often suggested (reducing the impression that they were unilateral foreign impositions). Nonetheless, in Ecuador, there was simply not a strong presence of the Foundation's International Health emissaries. Likely the fact that there were not large US-owned enterprises in the country was linked to relatively less Rockefeller Foundation activity to protect workers, ports, and generally US assets.

This book thus argues that international processes conditioned but did not determine how Ecuadorians defined or grappled with public health issues. Most importantly for the current purposes, public health campaigns were essentially national projects, carried out by cocitizens of the recipient population, although external assistance was recruited where possible. Rather than being characterized by a strong degree of influence from abroad, distinctive instead was the sharing of information and experiences across regional spaces in Ecuador, most importantly between Guayaquil and Quito. One of the striking characteristics of Ecuador in comparison to many other Latin American countries is the way its nineteenth- and twentieth-century history appears to be a tale of two cities. Highland Quito was the center of political power as the national capital but was increasingly surpassed by the port city Guayaquil as a center of economic power in the late nineteenth century. The regional relationship between coast and highlands, Guayaquil and Quito, was a defining feature of the Ecuadorian liberal period, as many political negotiations and conflicts were expressed in regional terms. When it came to the first decades of public health work, however, there was a considerable sharing of information and personnel between these cities, which also increasingly radiated out from these two poles as the movement of staff, equipment, materials, ideas, and regulations began to circulate around the national territory.[63]

As conationals of the population their programs targeted, public health leaders were particularly influential in forging new notions of state and society as they carried out their work. Because public health measures sometimes involved limiting individual freedoms in the name of a larger social good, Ecuadorian public health officials were actively involved in not only addressing health problems but also constructing notions of a national interest that might stand above or apart from local social relations. As the language of "above or apart" suggests, there were important spatial dimensions to these processes.[64] The chapters that follow explore how the service extended itself into new spaces both across the national territory and into domestic and intimate spheres.

Chapter Overview

The arrival of bubonic plague in Guayaquil in 1908 was the immediate catalyst for the establishment of the Ecuadorian Sanidad service later that year, so efforts to combat plague appropriately open the narrative of this book in chapter 1. It was not only in Ecuador that plague had a central role in the emergence of public health. As Paul Slack argues for fourteenth-century Europe, "most of what we understand by public health, its basic rationale and ideology, was first formulated in the context of plague."[65] Indeed, medieval Europe's plague experience motivated a fundamental conceptual shift: not only that public authorities should deal with the *consequences* of disease (that is, relieve and support the sick and bury the dead) but also that they had a responsibility to attack its causes and means of transmission and so mitigate its impact. Such actions, to protect the broader public, might well impose limitations on individual liberties. The third plague pandemic, during which the disease first reached the Americas, did not have the dramatic consequences anywhere of the second pandemic associated with the Black Death in Europe. The latter included staggering mortality rates that might reach 50 to 60 percent of the population of European cities in specific outbreaks. While mortality rates were much lower everywhere in early twentieth-century plague—and the local conditions, international context, and forms of scientific knowledge were also very different—in both eras plague motivated new conceptions of the state's role in protecting the population's health. In Ecuador, plague had a protagonist role in the development of public health infrastructure and aptly opens up a series of questions that are pursued subsequently in this book.[66]

Reflecting on Ecuador's plague experience, we can go on to articulate some of the novel ways that public health campaigns contributed to ways of thinking about the state's role. Chapter 2 picks up on threads introduced in chapter 1 and develops an analysis of how the state idea and the state system were advanced through public health. Specifically, it probes how the notion of public health as a necessary state activity was established alongside a related challenge facing public health leaders: What was the nature of the public health infrastructure, including personnel networks, that would allow it to implement and extend its programs? The chapter highlights the rapid process through which public health arose as a legitimate area of state activity, the challenges of coordinating and aligning the practices of diverse agents to produce effective health interventions, and how these contributed to notions of a state that was separate from society and of its agents as technical experts rather than political actors.

Chapters 3 and 4 examine how the Sanidad reached into new spaces in the highlands in two different contexts. After Guayaquil, the second city to receive permanent public health employees was the national capital Quito in 1914. Chapter 3 explores how Sanidad officials in Quito in the 1910s and 1920s took on a central role in an increasing range of negotiations between different social actors over infrastructure reforms and municipal services. By doing so, they simultaneously enabled the aspirations of a range of Quito residents to gain access to services, deepened their coordination with municipal actors, and heightened the visibility and legitimacy of their own activities. This facilitated the Sanidad's entrance into domestic contexts to influence quite intimate everyday practices.

As the Sanidad service extended its reach out into the provinces in the 1910s and thereafter, new challenges emerged in negotiating the authority of central state-appointed officials in local contexts. Chapter 4 explores these issues in Tungurahua province in the central highlands, where a new public health delegate was appointed in the provincial capital Ambato, as in other provinces, in 1926. As the Sanidad service took on new responsibilities at the provincial level to oversee a range of activities that had public health implications, the difficulties provincial delegates sometimes faced illuminate the importance of both interinstitutional and interpersonal relationships in advancing these projects in the context of ongoing structural challenges. Both chapters 3 and 4 highlight some of the spatial dimensions of extending public health programs, demonstrating at the same time how heavily health interventions relied on social processes.

Chapter 5 presents another element of Sanidad responsibilities that became increasingly important through the 1920s and 1930s: monitoring pharmacies and "professional defense" (that is, defending the rights of medical professionals to practice), two closely aligned activities. Pharmacies were physical and social spaces where the interests and projects of multiple stakeholder groups might cross, as prescribing drugs, preparing and dispensing drugs, and sale of these products created intersecting circles of social actors with shifting alliances and conflicts. Again here, as in the areas explored in chapters 3 and 4, the mediating role and position of the Sanidad was crucially important to how these often-fraught situations unfolded.

The chapters that follow provide diverse lenses through which the establishment and extension of public health projects can be observed. As an anthropological study, this book is centrally concerned with the changing shape of social relations that oriented and resulted from public health work, while also exploring the flow of historical events. Throughout, attention is drawn to how elements of a state idea and a state system mutually constituted each other through the active engagements of diverse social actors whose paths intersected in public health encounters. The book argues that public health work was not only about health but also constituted a central dimension of how the state was conjured in Ecuador.

Chapter 1

Encountering Plague, Plague Encounters

> Plague has a most pernicious past; a present that is bad; and a future that seems to say to civilized man, "Your money or your life." It is for man to say whether, in paying tribute to plague, it shall be a toll of lives or a tax in money, and if the latter, how much shall be paid and how payment shall be made.
>
> **—Dr. Bolívar Lloyd, 1925**

In February 1908, a plague outbreak was declared in Guayaquil, some five years after the disease first appeared down the Pacific coast in Callao and Lima, Peru. This chapter explores how Ecuador confronted plague, punctuated by extended discussion of two plague campaign "encounters" in the central highlands that illustrate the importance of the local circumstances within which public health projects unfolded. The shifting contours of plague outbreaks in regional spaces, moving between urban and rural locations and between coast and highlands, was an important dimension of Ecuador's experience with plague. These movements shaped both anti-plague campaigns and the structure of the public health service itself.

Situating Plague

For the first time, bubonic plague reached the Americas during the third pandemic of the disease.[1] After an outbreak in mainland China spread to Hong Kong in 1894, transmission gained considerable momentum. At the time, Hong Kong was the busiest port in the world, processing twenty-two million tons of goods annually (two million more than London).[2] Facilitated by steamship and railway links, plague reached across to the Americas, arriving in three separate events: a ship from Rotterdam brought it to Paraguay in April 1899 (later spreading to Argentina and Brazil); a ship likely carrying infected rice from Asia landed in San Francisco in 1900 (spreading infection subsequently to several other US cities and to Mexico); and a ship from Bangkok brought the plague to Peru in April 1903 (reaching Chile soon thereafter, and eventually Ecuador in February 1908). An ancient disease, plague's trajectory in the Americas was marked by modernity and economic integration operating on global, national, and regional scales.

Throughout the Americas, the number of confirmed plague cases up to 1938 was greatest in Peru (over 21,000 cases from 1903) and Ecuador (over 11,000 cases from 1908).[3] For purposes of comparison, in all of California, including the outbreaks in San Francisco, there were 372 cases from 1900 to 1925.[4] By 1923, in the Americas only Ecuador and Peru were considered significant plague areas with relatively high prevalence of the disease.[5] These two countries thus became focal points of anti-plague measures in the new world, involving both national campaigns and international cooperation. For instance, in 1929 traveling representative Dr. John Long, from the Pan American Sanitary Bureau (Oficina Sanitaria Pan Americana), and epidemiologist Dr. Clifford Eskey, from the US Public Health Service, arrived to work with Ecuadorian and Peruvian authorities to intensify anti-plague efforts in those countries. Plague was also one of four diseases (joining cholera, smallpox, and yellow fever after the 1897 International Sanitary Conference) that were of compulsory notification under international sanitary agreements, and whose existence could provoke strict quarantine measures affecting international trade. While plague was not the biggest killer in Ecuador, not even in Guayaquil where it claimed its largest number of victims,[6] the arrival of this dreaded disease alarmed the country and was the catalyst for the establishment of the Servicio de Sanidad (Public Health Service) a few months later.

The *Yersinia pestis* bacteria is usually found in small mammals, is transmitted between animals via their fleas, and as a zoonotic bacterium, can also transmit from animals to humans.[7] In other words, it is only incidentally a human disease.[8] The most common form of plague is bubonic plague, spread by fleas that feed on infected rodents and that, if the rodents die of plague, may seek out a human host for their next bloodmeal. In bubonic plague the typical lesions in humans are "buboes," or painful swellings that appear in the groin, armpit, and neck. In the Ecuadorian port of Guayaquil, mortality from bubonic plague was reported to be about 60 percent if it was untreated; under 35 percent if treated with *suero Yersin* (anti-plague serum developed by the Pasteur Institute, which boosted the immune system with blood serum); and 20 percent or less if treated with *suero Yersin* within twenty-four to thirty-six hours after onset, underlining the importance of early diagnosis.[9] Immunization with *linfa de Haffkine*—a vaccine that had been developed by Ukrainian bacteriologist Waldemar Haffkine during the 1897 outbreak in India—was, in contrast, a preventive measure. Other preventive measures focused on the elimination of rats and fleas; isolation of patients; disinfection of clothing and houses (or where disinfection was not possible, the burning of items and dwellings); and care in the transportation and disposal of cadavers.[10]

Another variant of the disease is septicemic plague, where the patient dies of sudden blood poisoning before the buboes have time to appear. An even more virulent form is pneumonic plague, which is spread directly from person to person by infected droplets in the breath; mortality is close to 100 percent, in part because cases are rarely recognized as such in a timely way. In Ecuador, after the transfer of a pneumonic plague patient from the Alausí area to the hospital in the provincial capital Riobamba in 1939, before plague was diagnosed, eleven nuns who staffed the hospital and Dr. Alfonso Villagómez (long-time provincial public health delegate) were infected and died within four days.[11] Finally, two rare forms of plague also appeared in Ecuador: *septicemia eruptiva* (*viruela pestosa*) and *angina pestosa*.[12] The former was characterized by the formation of pus-filled eruptions on the skin, the contents of which were highly contagious on touch, while the latter was a pharyngeal and tonsillar form of plague, with the growth of buboes in the throat that might lead to asphyxia. In both cases, mortality rates were well over 90 percent.

The microbe that causes plague was only identified in 1894, during the outbreak in Hong Kong. Prior to this identification, plague was a disease defined by its *symptoms*; afterwards, it was defined by the presence of a pathogen—that is, by its *cause*. While the symptoms of the main varieties of plague are different, what is common to them all is the presence of the plague pathogen, *Yersinia pestis*, something that can only be determined in a laboratory.[13] Identification of the plague microbe did not however reveal how the organism was transmitted; during the following decade, the role of rats in the spread of plague was identified. When the Second International Sanitary Conference of the Americas met in Washington in 1905, they agreed to anti-plague measures that focused on rats, but they did not yet target an insect vector.[14] In the early years of the twentieth century, rat fleas were discovered to be the actual transmitters of plague, but it took additional time to understand why the biting rat flea *Xenopsylla cheopis* was the most efficient in transmitting plague. Not only is it parasitic on the main victims of plague (black rats), but the shape of its proventriculus causes the latter to become blocked by bacilli when the flea feeds on infected blood, which it regurgitates into the next host it bites.

When considering Ecuador's experience with plague in the early twentieth century, one must remember that research was ongoing into the causes of the disease and that the complex connections among different factors influencing disease ecology had not yet been untangled. Medical entomology did not keep up with the advances in identification of disease microorganisms, and debate was ongoing about whether there was an insect vector (and if so, which insect). Plague ecology itself varied in different contexts, with diverse rodents serving as reservoirs: while rats are the most common carriers of plague, it also infected prairie dogs and ground squirrels in the southwestern United States, gerbils in South Africa, marmots in Manchuria, and as Ecuadorians found out, guinea pigs. Even once rats and their fleas were identified as key players in plague transmission, preventive measures might have unintended consequences. Energetic disinfection campaigns could drive rats out of their shelters and into closer contact with humans; massive rat kills during outbreaks could force hungry fleas to search out new hosts.[15] While laboratory *identification* of plague in the early twentieth century was relatively easy—as long as appropriate facilities were available—*preventing* the disease was much more difficult. Effective *treatment* was even more elusive. In 1954, the World Health Organization (WHO) stated, "It is only within the last decade that treatment with sulfonamides and antibiotics, on the one hand, and the application of potent pesticides—particularly DDT—on the other, have rendered plague both a normally curable and a thoroughly controllable disease."[16] Nonetheless, since 1996 WHO has classified plague as a reemerging disease. A quarter century later, WHO identifies the Democratic Republic of Congo, Madagascar, and Peru as three countries that have ongoing problems with plague outbreaks.[17]

Thus, when plague arrived in Guayaquil, Ecuador, in early 1908, the laboratory identification of the pathogen was relatively recent, and many questions remained about plague transmission. The first plague victims were dock and customs house workers in the port, along with city residents who frequented the nearby public market.[18] Following 63 human cases in February 1908, there were 225 cases in March, the greatest number ever reported in Guayaquil for a single month. In 1909, the inland towns of Yaguachi, Milagro, and Huigra along the railway line were invaded by plague, signaled first by epizootics among rats in the railway stations, followed by human cases among those who worked in the vicinity. In an unfortunate historical coincidence, the Guayaquil-Quito Railway was nearing completion to Quito when plague arrived in Guayaquil. Inaugurated in June 1908, the railway linked the port with the

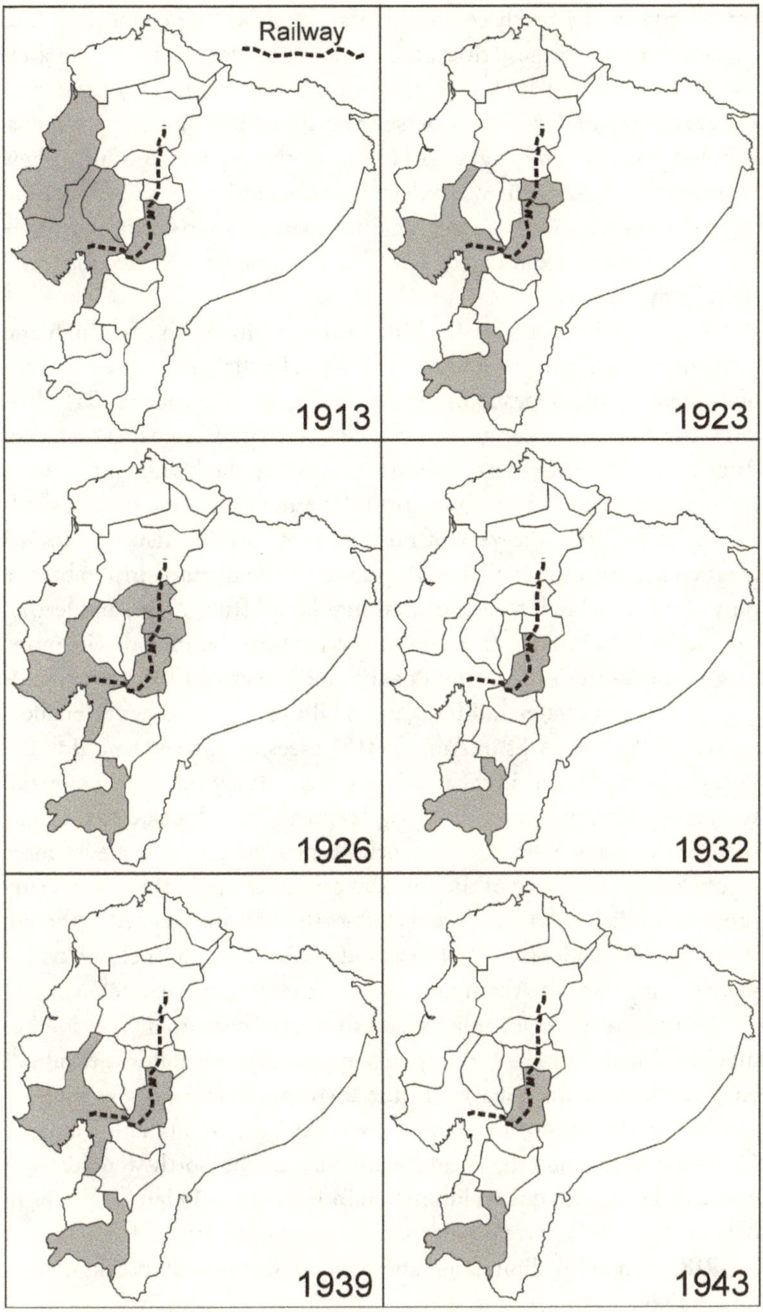

Map 2. Plague outbreaks in Ecuadorian provinces, selected dates. Plague was present continuously in Ecuador from 1908, when it first infected Guayas province, through the 1940s. These maps present key changes in the extension of plague across provinces. ***Credit:*** **Edward Eastaugh.**

capital city in the north-central highlands, altogether connecting four of Ecuador's five largest cities; only Cuenca in the southern highlands was far from the railway line. Plague spread along the railway route from the port to the highland interior (see map 2). Riding on railway wagons, infected rats brought plague to Huigra in the Andean foothills a few months after Guayaquil was infected, attracted by the railway station storehouses for staple foods awaiting transport south to Cuenca by muleback. Plague never did invade Cuenca, given rats' preference for travel on railway wagons.

Plague arrived in Alausí, Chimborazo province—the first highland town infected, northeast and up the mountains from Huigra—in 1913 and spread up the slopes to Indigenous villages of the zone in 1914. That year, the Sanidad accurately identified the city of Ambato, capital of Tungurahua province north of Chimborazo, as the highland city most likely to be invaded by plague, given "the multiplication of thousands of rats."[19] In 1916, the year of greatest virulence in Alausí (with 167 plague cases in this small town), plague was confirmed in Ambato, a busy commercial hub for the central highlands' fruit, grain, and leather production. As in Alausí, so too in the next canton inland, Guamote, plague spread from the vicinity of the rail line after 1918 to surrounding agricultural estates and Indigenous villages. In 1926, with the most serious of the outbreaks in Ambato (101 cases), plague advanced to the village of Guaytacama in the province of León (later renamed Cotopaxi) to the north. Similarly, in 1929, plague spread from Ambato to the rural outskirts of Latacunga, the provincial capital of León, located a mere eighty kilometers south of the national capital Quito in the neighboring province of Pichincha. This was as far north as plague reached, although it was not self-evident that Quito would not be infected. A closer look at plague campaigns in Alausí and Guaytacama is presented below.

In the coastal region, plague spread by riverboat from Guayaquil to inland Babahoyo in 1909, with yearly appearances until it was eliminated in 1918. South of Guayaquil, the town of Santa Rosa was infected in 1911, with elimination in 1918. The ports of Manta and Bahía de Caráquez in neighboring Manabí province to the north were also invaded in 1913, with quick elimination in Bahía in 1914 but outbreaks in Manta until 1916. Several other smaller towns in Manabí were infected in 1918, with rapid elimination and only a few minor outbreaks ending in the 1920s in this region.

In southern Ecuador, plague crossed to Loja province not from elsewhere in Ecuador but from northern Peru, with the first infection in 1921. The Loja outbreaks were important in their own right but were not seen as a threat to other parts of the national territory, since the province was relatively isolated from the remainder of the country by topography; in contrast, it was in intensive contact with northern Peru. Ultimately, the areas where plague established a more secure foothold were in urban Guayaquil and in rural areas in the central highland province of Chimborazo and in southern Loja province bordering Peru. While the Guayaquil outbreaks shared characteristics typical of urban plague elsewhere, the latter two regions had different experiences with what came to be known as sylvatic or rural plague.

Plague represented an enormous challenge for Ecuadorian public health. A disease such as hookworm could be both treated and prevented relatively easily, not only improving people's health but vividly illustrating the value of medical and public health measures.[20] Yellow fever, in turn, was limited to the range of the *Aedes aegypti* mosquito, conferred some immunity on those who recovered, and in the absence of fundamental reform of water supply systems, could still be dealt with in urban areas by disrupting the reproductive cycle of mosquitoes. Plague, however, was especially difficult to control. Rats themselves are resilient creatures that reproduce rapidly: if only a single pair of rats remained in an extirpation campaign, under favorable conditions this pair would be capable of producing four hundred to six hundred rats within a period of fifteen to eighteen months.[21] Plague caused fear, illness, and death in Ecuador and strained the resources and challenged the personnel of the Sanidad. It also had a considerable impact on the structure and development of the public health service, and hence Ecuador's plague experience opens up many of the questions pursued in this book.

Early Plague Campaigns in Ecuador

"Rats are dying in large numbers all over the city of Guayaquil. Sick rats are often seen in broad daylight. In accordance with instructions from President Alfaro, I have been tendered the laboratories of the Colegio Vicente Rocafuerte, and two prominent physicians have been named to cooperate with me in the bacteriological examinations."[22] Thus reported US physician and consular official Dr. Bolívar Lloyd from Guayaquil on February 11, 1908; laboratory identification was confirmed on February 25 and the port city was officially declared infected.[23] Lloyd's comments point to ways that Ecuador was ill prepared, in terms of institutional infrastructure, to meet a significant new health threat. In February 1908 there was no national government agency in Ecuador that was charged with overseeing public health. Rather, in the port there was a working group of municipal officials, police, physicians, and port authorities who together formed a local board of health. As assistant surgeon of the

United States Public Health and Marine-Hospital Service, Lloyd was charged with inspecting ships and signing bills of health for any vessels in the Guayaquil port that were bound for ports in the US or Panama.[24] He led the laboratory identification of plague using the municipal equipment that had recently been installed at the men's high school.[25] Lloyd was then appointed director of a special commission established in late March to deal with the plague threat. This commission was replaced in November by the Ecuadorian Servicio de Sanidad, established by Congress.

In the early twentieth century, with limited treatment options, Ecuadorian officials emphasized containment over care in their plague campaigns. Anti-plague work in Guayaquil was conducted on three main fronts, piloting the measures that would be used elsewhere in the country. There were efforts to eliminate rats in the city via rat catching or poisoning, reduction of their nesting areas through a transformation of urban architecture, and increased control over garbage disposal; other measures targeted control of commerce and transportation in an effort to prevent the spread of plague to the highlands; and the ill were isolated and any contaminated possessions and dwellings disinfected. Guayaquil's urban architecture lent itself to rat nests, providing harborage in the interior of double-wall constructions in wooden buildings or in the decorative material boxing in exterior columns. While it was possible to ensure that new buildings and houses were constructed with rat-proofing measures (and new architectural codes were developed in response to plague to ensure this), it was more difficult and expensive to reduce rat harborage in older buildings. However, the periodic fires that swept through Guayaquil made the replacement of some of its older wooden buildings unavoidable.

From the arrival of plague in Guayaquil in 1908 until it was first eliminated in the port in 1930, important elements of the anti-plague campaign focused on the control of trade and transportation. Commercial interests were of fundamental importance to the anti-plague campaigns, in terms of the port's relation with the exterior: outbreaks could cause the port to be boycotted by international steamship lines. Commercial and transportation links within the country were also a principal cause of the spread of plague from one locale to another. Train cargo was fumigated in a vain effort to prevent rats from traveling on the cargo wagons. These efforts were frustrated by the fact that the railway company was using open cages intended for moving livestock as its cargo wagons for the transport of merchandise,[26] which made it impossible to fumigate them effectively. Railway station architecture was also problematic. In March 1916 the railway company's limited offer to refill the floors of the railway warehouses was considered insufficient: the Sanidad insisted that all double wall constructions should be replaced with either single walls or solid material, and the wooden floors of the main railway installations should be replaced with solid, impermeable material, preferably cement. Only major renovations would eliminate rat harborage.

There was also attention to monitoring train passengers traveling in either direction between the port and the highlands to ensure that they were first immunized with Haffkine's vaccine. Targeted vaccination of travelers and of residents in outbreak zones was prioritized over a broader vaccination program, given limited vaccine supplies. The mechanisms to monitor train passengers' status were varied: for instance, in 1913 and 1914 passports to enable internal travel were issued by the police to those who showed proof of having been vaccinated, and similarly, railway employees were prohibited from selling tickets to those without vaccination certificates. In November 1914 a vaccination office was established in the northern railway terminus in Chimbacalle (on the outskirts of Quito), so that there would be no excuse for passengers to embark for the coast without having been vaccinated. However, in the provincial city Ambato, in a seven-week period in mid-1916, fifteen train passengers were discovered to be carrying falsified vaccination certificates and seventy-four more presented certificates belonging to others; there were also ninety-six train passengers who were prevented from traveling due to lack of vaccination certificates.[27] While this indicates some success in monitoring vaccination status, it also reveals many attempts to evade the measures of control. The Sanidad itself was having difficulty obtaining enough vaccine from a laboratory in Lima, which interfered with its efforts to ensure vaccination.[28]

The isolation of the ill, long a staple of plague prevention, was also essential to reduce the spread of plague. However, the state of Ecuadorian quarantine facilities led wealthy and poor residents alike to avoid them whenever possible. In Guayaquil, a special lazaretto was in service by the mid-1910s with improved conditions for paying patients; this *lazareto de pensionados* was also used for yellow fever patients when plague subsided seasonally, since at the time there was no such improved facility available for their isolation. Compulsory quarantine in isolation hospitals was controversial, even among physicians. In the face of some physicians' skepticism, Sanidad director general Dr. León Becerra commented wearily to the Quito subdirector in 1917 that even in the most advanced countries one could find scientific celebrities who denied the measures that science and experience dictated.[29] Along with isolation of the ill themselves, their possessions and dwellings were disinfected to prevent the spread of disease. However, given that only some kinds of architecture could be disinfected, housing with features such as straw roofs was more likely to be burned to eliminate the insect vector, disproportionately affecting the poor.

When the initial highland plague outbreaks occurred in 1913 and 1914 in Alausí, Chimborazo province[30]—the first Andean town on the railway's route inland from the coast—the Sanidad campaign revealed both general features and others specific to local social relations, meriting a closer look. The anti-plague measures were led by Sanidad staff from Guayaquil, the only city with permanent public health employees, who applied in Alausí approaches they had used in the port. These focused on the elimination of sources of infection and the vaccination of the healthy. A rat-hunting team was set up that killed 1,445 rats in the town in April 1913 alone; wherever infected rats were found, streets and houses were chemically disinfected; double-wall constructions in houses and the railway station were destroyed; domestic animals were poisoned or driven out of the town limits; infected people were quarantined in a rapidly built isolation hut to which alarmed townspeople contributed funding; and the area's inhabitants were subject to an obligatory vaccination campaign (for instance, 1,032 people in the town center were vaccinated in April 1913[31]). The campaign was financed by the national government—Alausí was the only highland town that received any funding for public health from the national treasury in 1913—supplemented by the meager municipal budget.

Given the lack of any local infrastructure or personnel for carrying out a public health campaign of this kind, mechanisms were used that had a long history in this area. The municipal police recruited day laborers to do much of the work of disinfection and garbage disposal, activating the same procedures they had been using for many years to recruit labor for municipal public works. They forcibly recruited laborers—working with the cantonal political administrator to engage parish-level political lieutenants in this effort—from among adult Indigenous men living in the surrounding peasant communities. Indigenous day laborers in this zone had a history of actively contesting forced labor recruitment by municipal authorities and had achieved a number of victories against local abuses in this arena in previous years, often with support from central government officials.[32] Their petitions were consistent with ways that liberal officials emphasized fundamental rights to enter freely into labor contracts, rhetoric that local Indigenous leaders adeptly repeated back to state officials. While a discourse about race was not clearly articulated, the recruitment practices themselves were racialized in their focus on Indigenous workers. It is notable that anti-plague work was the only area in which new labor demands were imposed in the 1910s and where central government officials were unresponsive to Indigenous complaints about abuses of their constitutional rights. In this case, stopping plague from spreading further inland was a greater priority for the national government than its emphasis in other situations on liberalizing labor conditions in the highlands (ultimately to free labor for migrations to agro-export zones on the coast) or enhancing central government control over local officials. The latter were both central features of liberal government practices (pursued in stops and starts) in the first decades of the twentieth century. It is likely that the form of labor recruitment itself had unfortunate consequences beyond the local population: it is plausible that it was when Indigenous peasants were forced to work in plague zones that they carried the contagion back into their communities, where it became very difficult indeed to eliminate.

Anti-plague work in Alausí had to grapple with not only complex social dynamics but also funding challenges. In March 1916, with the first plague outbreak in Ambato that was traced back to new cases in Alausí, the public health service was able to pay the salary of a licentiate in medicine who was sent from Guayaquil to Alausí to carry out anti-plague work. However, there was only the insufficient quantity of 60 sucres per month (about 30 dollars at the exchange rate of the time) from the Alausí municipal coffers to pay for all other expenses associated with the campaign, including costs of transportation, labor, supplies, and food for patients isolated in the lazaretto. The service estimated that some 3,000 sucres were needed to conduct a sufficiently rapid and energetic campaign in Alausí to save the interior provinces. Luckily the *licenciado* was accompanied by two colleagues who were willing to go along for the experience ("*por el amor al arte*") and without compensation. The government did approve 1,000 sucres in extraordinary funds for the sanitation of Alausí, enough to finance one month's work. The commission in Alausí proceeded "to burn down various houses, kill hundreds of *cuyes* [guinea pigs], vaccinate more than 100 people (with vaccine for 500 more on the way), obligate the inhabitants to keep houses and streets clean, monitor passengers, and fumigate cargo,"[33] only to discover that the provincial treasurer in Riobamba who was to reimburse these expenditures claimed that the treasury was empty. Later that year the national government earmarked 300 sucres per month to fight plague in Alausí, but again there was difficulty in getting access to even those modest funds. In February 1917, the service withdrew its campaign in Alausí given the lack of funds to continue it, even though it was coming up to the season when plague normally reappeared in the area.

Meanwhile in Quito, when plague crept up the rail line from Guayaquil to Alausí in April 1913, in the absence of a public health office in the capital, the minister of the interior gathered together prominent Quito physicians (none of whom had experience fighting plague) to meet with him to develop a series of anti-plague measures to protect the highland cities. The recommended measures covered examination of train passengers and their baggage in Riobamba, Ambato, and Latacunga (the capitals of the three highland provinces between Guayas and Pichincha), provision of serum and vaccine to physicians in those cities, verification of vaccination status of travelers, and establishment of lazarettos for plague patients in provincial capitals and Quito. What is most striking, however, is the lack of clear lines of authority and of personnel networks to deal with a public health threat of this kind (issues further explored in the next chapter). The physicians of the capital agreed to meet three times a week in the minister's office to monitor the situation, indicating the urgency of the circumstances. They resolved among other things to urge the municipal councils of Riobamba, Ambato and Latacunga to appoint *médicos de higiene*—rather than simply *municipal physicians* with a wide range of responsibilities[34]—who would be able to carry out the kinds of monitoring they recommended. The content of their resolutions was passed on to the director of the Junta de Sanidad e Higiene in Quito, by means of the governor of the province, copying to the director the memorandum that the governor had received from the minister, in a laboriously retyped series of memos (each of which transcribed the previous ones). Despite the evident need to be able to transmit orders to more local instances of government, the minister argued a few months later in his annual report that "the autonomy of the [Municipal] Councils is, to my mind, the sine qua non for the progress of the cantons."[35] The contradiction between these two issues suggests the uneasy relations between officials positioned at different scales. As it turned out, even in the capital in April 1913 it was difficult to ensure cooperation: the president of the municipal council of Quito felt compelled to express his regrets to the municipal director of hygiene for the difficulties he was experiencing and urged him not to give up on his important anti-plague measures, carried out in the capital with minimal funds and even less public support.[36]

It was in this context that a few months later in August 1913, Dr. Carlos Miño, who had overseen the plague campaign in Alausí in April, was named a delegate of the Guayaquil central Sanidad office in the capital Quito; his status was elevated to regional subdirector effective January 1914.[37] This made the capital and the port the only two cities in Ecuador with permanently stationed public health employees appointed and funded by the national government. The arrival of an experienced public health physician enabled a more coordinated and wide-ranging campaign to address infectious disease threats. In Quito, the perceived danger of plague infection likely facilitated Miño's energetic domestic inspection program (see chapter 3). In extreme cases, Quito's sanitary regulation also authorized the closure (*clausura*) of properties to enforce public health measures. The most significant achievement in this regard was the closure and demolition of the railway station in Chimbacalle, following several years of conflicts over its sanitary conditions.[38] A new facility was inaugurated on the May 24 civic holiday in 1920. While having a direct positive impact on the plague threat, this undoubtedly also constituted a public relations triumph for the Sanidad. As Miño comments, "the subdirectorate took on the task of obligating the Company to demolish that poor, ugly, repugnant rats' nest ironically called a Station, and to substitute for it a suitable building in harmony with the advance of the city and above all with the interests of public health."[39]

In Quito, Miño promoted a broad program of sanitary reforms, perhaps taking advantage of a sense of urgency to encourage general changes to behavior that public health reformers were sure would have preventive health benefits. Thus, a broadsheet was published in June 1916 tying a wide range of measures of household and individual hygiene to the prevention of plague. Institutional measures focused on monitoring travelers and cargo arriving in Quito from the south. Residents, however, could also do their part through reforming household hygiene: they were urged to maintain scrupulous cleanliness in their habitations, sweeping them daily and using a disinfectant, and to air out their lodgings, leaving windows and doors open for as many hours a day as possible since "the plague bacillus does not like solar light, above all direct light that kills it quickly. It is therefore beneficial that light and air penetrate amply the habitations since these are the most powerful natural disinfectants." Moreover, they should not keep domestic animals in their rooms, especially cuyes; they should use all means to destroy rats and mice, who under the circumstances were "the worst enemies of man"; they should use whatever means were available to destroy fleas, which transmitted plague if they had fed on infected rats or mice; and they should collect household garbage in covered metallic containers to deprive rats of their daily food. Property owners—for their own security—were further authorized to inspect their tenants' lodgings and to destroy any domestic pigs, cuyes, or rabbits kept within the urban area. In terms of individual hygiene, people were advised to observe the most rigorous personal cleanliness, bathing frequently and changing their underwear at least twice a week. "Plague preferentially attacks dirty people and thus the most scrupulous personal and household cleanliness is necessary." Moreover, people should "use the greatest regularity and moderation in food, drink, and all of life's acts. They should exclude from their alimentation substances that are irritants or difficult to digest, unripe fruit, and in general, poorly cooked foods."[40] This document included both clear statements about how plague was spread specifically by fleas that had fed on infected rats and general suggestions for personal hygiene and behavior in support of preventive health campaigns. Miño's reference to dirty people does not seem to be class-specific, given other elements of his program in Quito (chapter 3) that palpably included altering the behavior of wealthier residents.

In September 1917 there was also an intensification of rat catching in the capital, with the division of the city into five zones for this work and a public health inspector and peon assigned to each one to place traps and distribute poison. Their reports indicate a great increase in the specificity and detail of the Sanidad's understanding of the timing and trajectory of the arrival and movement of rats from building to building along key streets in the capital.[41] Their intensive efforts in the streets of the capital, drawing on residents' observations of the spread of rats via a door-to-door survey, would have also elevated public awareness of the service's activities. This work highlights an essential feature of Sanidad activities: gathering and systematizing information.

While the Sanidad was working to strengthen its personnel networks for addressing public health threats in the mid-1910s, it did so in an era marked by considerable financial constraints. Those years saw a civil war fought in the northern coast region as well as disruption of international trade due to the First World War, both of which impacted the financial resources available to fight plague. Effective February 1915 the Sanidad had its monthly funding cut in half, just at a time that it needed to expand its services with the spread of plague toward the interior of the country. The reduced monthly budget of 10,000 sucres for the whole service meant that anti-plague expenditures were limited to paying the employees of the lazarettos in Durán (the railway terminus across the Guayas River from Guayaquil), Huigra, and Alausí, since these locations were considered the possible transmission points of plague toward the interior.[42] By April 1915, funding for preventive measures for all public health purposes was eliminated. When plague reappeared in Alausí in May, there were not even funds to send a squad of workers and a physician to the area. When plague resurfaced in Guayaquil in late July, the only measure available was vaccination since there were no funds for other supplies. Still, to immunize twenty thousand people would cost 4,000 sucres, without considering the salaries of the vaccinators (who were themselves scarce).[43] As public health officials knew very well, vaccination could only be obligatory if it was free of charge.

Another obstacle to anti-plague campaigns was some ongoing skepticism about how plague was transmitted. As Miño felt compelled to explain to the cabinet minister responsible for the public health portfolio in 1916:

> It is fully proven not only in this country but in others that have been invaded by plague that the true and most efficient transmitter of the plague bacillus is not man but rodents, and especially the rat, given its living conditions and adaptability to all climates and conditions. That the rat is the true transmitter, has been demonstrated in Huigra, the first of the towns along the railway line to be infected, and then subsequently in Alausí and Ambato and other locations where cargo wagons are gathered. Another proof is that Riobamba, where the cargo trains do not enter, has not been infected, despite having received a person infected with plague and being the obligatory stop for all passengers from the north and south on the railway line.[44] If Huigra was infected before Milagro, Naranjito and Yaguachi, it is because it is the cargo station for the provinces to the south of the republic. On the other hand, in no location has the plague appeared first among human victims, but rather infallibly the epizooty.[45]

Despite the Sanidad's efforts to combat plague outbreaks, to reform living conditions that might facilitate plague infection in the first place, and generally to persuade political leaders and the broader population about the nature of the threat, back in Guayaquil when the disease seasonally reappeared the service was often berated in the press. Miño sympathized with the difficulties faced by Director General Becerra in Guayaquil, who bore the brunt of such attacks. As Miño comments, "The government has no problem emitting decrees that are impossible to fulfill given the lack of funds; with these decrees the government washes its hands before the public and you [Becerra] will no doubt be the Christ [that is, crucified] when the public demands services that cannot possibly be provided due to the absolute lack of resources."[46] Yet again, the media campaign was renewed at the end of 1920, with the reappearance of plague in Guayaquil. Becerra knew very well the challenges they faced:

> For the plague to disappear it would be necessary to undertake reforms well beyond the country's means. Millions would be necessary to change the old construction of Guayaquil's buildings, and cleanse the ground with drainage, sewage, and paving of its streets. That is the only way we will be free of the rats that are vectors of this fatal disease. The Sanidad fights with the few resources it is granted, achieving miracles to attend to the many services demanded of it, without support of the municipality and overcoming the resistance of the residents. To ask the government for more

> resources would be pure stubbornness on my part, since I am well aware of the penury of the state, and I know the many struggles faced by the patriot who is leading the national government.[47]

In the face of the press campaign, Becerra determined to resign, but events seem to have overtaken his decision: he died five days after sharing these thoughts with Miño. The government then named Dr. Wenceslao Pareja to the director general position, promoting him from his role as the service's physician overseeing Guayaquil's three lazarettos (for plague, yellow fever, and smallpox). Pareja apparently had the confidence of the municipal council of Guayaquil, who at his request entrusted the Sanidad with the garbage collection and disposal service in the port city. This was a challenging responsibility, to be sure, but in Pareja's view was a necessary first step in his larger plan to eliminate plague.[48] Pareja credited this dual approach of using targeted measures to combat specific outbreaks along with a more general hygienization of the city for the low figure of plague cases in the port in 1922: for the first time since 1908 the annual number dropped below 200, amounting to only 56 cases in 1922 compared to 270 the previous year.[49]

When plague reappeared in Ambato in October 1923, it created another opportunity for the Sanidad to insist on the need to establish permanent campaigns to combat diseases as well as to remove their preconditions—in the case of plague, especially in those areas (such as Ambato and Alausí) where large supplies of foodstuffs were stored because they were nodal points in trade networks. The plague was likened to an oil spill, "spreading slowly but inexorably, permanent and persistent, requiring constant and energetic measures in infected areas."[50] Since plague persisted in Guayaquil, and the port was in continual and increasing communication with the interior, the possibility that plague would invade and become permanent in the highland cities haunted public health officials.

Reorganization and Coordination

On July 9, 1925, a bloodless coup, the Revolución Juliana, brought to an end three decades dominated politically by the Liberal Party. This initiated a period of centralization and coordination of government institutions in general, including for public health. Consistent with the consolidation of other government institutions in Quito after the Juliana, the Sanidad main office was moved to Quito, and a new subdirector position was created for the southern zone headquartered in Cuenca, in addition to the subdirector in Guayaquil for the coastal provinces. By early 1926, the new director general of Sanidad (who served simultaneously as subdirector of the north-central zone) was physician Pablo Arturo Suárez, whose own areas of expertise were tuberculosis and social medicine more generally. From April to July 1926, first in zones affected by plague and then in other provincial capitals, provincial delegates of Sanidad were finally established who reported to the regional subdirectors for each zone and through them to the director general in Quito.

This period also saw increased international cooperation, observable in the 1929 arrival of the American Commission. But already in September 1926 Suárez had taken advantage of his visit to Washington for the First Pan American Conference of Public Health Directors (discussed further in chapter 2) to form part of a three-person commission to formulate a plan of research into plague to be carried out by public health officials in affected countries in the Americas. This plan focused especially on the detailed study of rat and flea populations (including identification of species of rodents and fleas, sex and age of rats correlated with intensity of flea infestations, and several other variables) to clarify the nature of transmission in order to better design preventive measures. The commission hoped that sufficient comparative data, if systematically collected, would help them unravel continuing uncertainties about plague, such that detailed "surveys . . . if made by a considerable number of countries over a period of at least one year under identical circumstances, with records of results that are strictly comparable, will serve more definitely to fix upon the exact species and quantities of rodents and ecto-parasites that make possible the propagation of plague."[51]

During this trip, Suárez spent several days at Rosebank Quarantine Station in New York being trained by entomologists in the techniques used there to classify flea species. Based on the program developed by the commission, public health employees in various countries in the Americas proceeded to trap, kill, and autopsy rats and collect, count, and classify the fleas of rodents in order to contribute to the growing body of knowledge about plague transmission. Ecuador was the first country in Latin America to initiate these studies, as rat catchers and technicians trapped rats, collected fleas, and analyzed species of fleas that "predominantly," "occasionally," and "rarely" affected different rodent species. Indeed, a representative of the Pan American Sanitary Bureau singled out the Ecuadorian investigation as providing a model for other nations given its rigorous methodology. Already by early December 1926 Suárez had extended this research to the highlands and could confirm the role of the *cheopis* flea in the propagation of plague: the only highland locations where this flea was found were in those regularly infected with plague, such as Ambato and Alausí. The *cheopis* flea was normally not found on human beings or on any animals other than rats and had not been encountered in Quito.[52] One way that Suárez's leadership in this area was recognized was that a new species of flea discovered during this research was named for him, *Hectopsylla suarez*. The work of Ecuadorian public health physicians and their teams could appropriately be seen as an example of "scientific excellence in the periphery," a phenomenon highlighted by historian Marcos Cueto.[53]

While in urban locations such as Guayaquil and Ambato the role of rats in spreading plague was clear, the newly appointed Sanidad delegates in the central highland provinces of Tungurahua and León were less certain in 1926 about how plague spread in rural areas. Early on—even before his trip to Washington—Suárez instructed them to begin to examine the kinds of fleas carried by cuyes and other domesticated animals and rodents in rural areas, since he had already begun to explore plague transmission in areas without rats. From April to July 1926 (immediately upon taking up his position), the new delegate in Chimborazo initiated anti-plague campaigns in various rural areas of the province and, foreshadowing future patterns, noted the "special circumstance that all of the plague cases have occurred among Indigenous people."[54] Indeed, it was becoming increasingly apparent that plague was not only an urban phenomenon associated with rats but also beginning to appear in rural areas under quite different circumstances that might require a modified approach to eradication.

In May 1926 plague broke out in Guaytacama, a rural zone of León province.[55] The evolving profile of public health work can be seen in the service's response, although as in Alausí the local specificities also merit attention. Guaytacama was the location of several large modernizing agricultural estates (*haciendas*) that had otherwise benefited from the construction of the railway through the area—especially for the intensification of dairy production to provision urban markets[56]—and whose busy trade with the port was indeed likely implicated in the zone's plague outbreak. In order to fight plague, a handful of influential large landowners of the zone—including Enrique Gangotena Jijón (who had been the president of the modernizing Sociedad Nacional de Agricultura[57] in the 1910s) and former national president Leonidas Plaza Gutiérrez (of coastal origins, but who had married into the Lasso family, prominent agriculturalists in this region)—together contributed several thousand sucres toward the anti-plague campaign, to fund the purchase of supplies and the costs of labor and mobilization associated with the measures.[58] They also formally agreed that their hacienda administrators would ensure cooperation with the vaccination and disinfection teams among the Indigenous peasants living on their estates. The direct involvement of large landowners and their administrators in the plague response sets this outbreak apart not just from urban but also from other rural ones. In Alausí, for instance, the key relations were instead between local government officials and independent Indigenous communities that did not live within the boundaries of large estates.

Dr. Pedro Zambrano was sent from Quito to oversee the Guaytacama campaign against plague. A young physician with an interest in social medicine, he had completed his thesis a few years earlier on the medical and social problems associated with prostitution in Quito (he went on to direct the Sanidad's Venereal Prophylaxis Service in Quito for many years[59]). In several instances, Zambrano showed an unusual sensitivity to the situation of the local population during the anti-plague campaign. He empathized with local Indigenous peons, who avoided work on the campaign due to fears of being infected—"as happened with the day worker Hualpa, who perished of plague on completing a fortnight's work; the product of his labor allowed his grandmother to buy him a coffin"[60]—and reduced recruitment for such squads. Then one night two subaltern employees at the lazaretto got drunk, locked the other employees in the bunk room, and attempted to sexually assault two Indigenous female plague patients in the lazaretto. Zambrano immediately contacted the provincial public health delegate to send police troops to arrest the perpetrators, and when the lazaretto employees were released from the Latacunga provincial jail a few days later, he protested strongly that such an abuse could not go unpunished. While his reports make clear that he was partly concerned with the pragmatic problem of gaining the trust of the Indigenous population, he also characterized this incident as having sickened his spirit.

Around the same time, a set of vaccines used in the campaign turned out to be adulterated, so that both vaccinated and unvaccinated alike died of plague, leading peasants to hide from the vaccinators. Zambrano observed that "the Indians are, like never before, completely pessimistic; they believe, and no one can convince them otherwise, that the vaccine is a poison that they are injected with in order to kill them."[61] Zambrano dedicated considerable time to investigating how the shipment was damaged, but he was unsuccessful. The following month an Indigenous uprising occurred (apparently provoked in part by the anti-plague campaign), and in its aftermath participants fled to distant communities. Zambrano's main concern was that the contagion might be spread, and so he provided certificates to Indigenous peasants confirming their innocence in the uprising to encourage them, successfully, to return to their communities.[62] The provincial Sanidad delegate in Latacunga joined him in urging that an order of release be issued to free the jailed leaders of the uprising, to respect an offer the public health official had made to them immediately after the incident.[63]

There are some striking elements in these accounts, such as the unusual mention *by name* of an Indigenous day laborer who had died of plague and the reference to Indigenous peasants as "pessimistic" rather than ignorant regarding the effects of vaccination. Contrasting with the sympathy shown for those groups, the director general requested legal sanctions against a large landowner who had repeatedly tried to recruit agricultural workers from an infected zone despite the *cordon sanitaire*.[64] He also went straight to President Isidro Ayora with his request for punishment of the *jefe político* (political administrator) of Salcedo canton and the *teniente político* (political lieutenant) of Saquisilí parish, who he argued held direct responsibility for having permitted religious fiestas to occur in their jurisdictions despite the plague threat; he also blamed the governor of the province for having neglected to prevent this.[65] In other words, Sanidad officials showed a significantly more punitive attitude toward people in positions of relative power who undermined the anti-plague campaign than they did toward Indigenous peasants who they seemed to recognize as victims with understandable concerns.

While containment was the goal of this campaign given limited treatment options, there were nonetheless significant elements of care, broadly defined. Where this was lacking, the results could be a failure of containment as well. In the outskirts of Ambato in 1926, for instance, the new provincial delegate reported that "in the hamlet 'Llallacha,' jurisdiction of Picaihua, where some cases of plague appeared, it was necessary to incinerate five straw huts because there was no other way of cleansing them. This circumstance and the incineration of clothing and old objects (*trastos viejos*) led, unfortunately, a large part of the population to flee, leaving their huts empty and taking themselves and their belongings to other places, thus propagating the terrible epidemic."[66] Working to establish relations of trust (or failing to do so) could have a significant impact on the spread of disease.

Both in rural areas of the central highlands and among poor urban inhabitants of Ambato, Suárez insisted in February 1927 on the importance of reforming sleeping conditions in dwellings. Based on research during the 1926 Guaytacama campaign, he developed a regulation requiring that people sleep on raised platforms rather than directly on the ground, to distance themselves from the fleas harbored by domestic animals as well as by rats that tended to enter huts at night in search of food (in rural areas rats generally lived outside, unlike in the crowded wooden tenements of Guayaquil).[67] He was inflexible regarding the importance of this measure but recognized the financial barriers and offered to provide one or two sucres per household to those who were unable to otherwise afford these *tarimas*; he also circulated instructions for their simple and economical construction. For the first time, Suárez also developed architectural norms for peasant huts (*chozas*) in the Andean countryside, emphasizing that they should have concrete foundations to avoid providing nesting places for burrowing rodents. These were difficult to enforce for economic reasons, but the Sanidad did finance the construction of a model hut to replace one that had been burned in the Guaytacama campaign. For the first time, too, the service paid compensation to peasants in the area whose huts had been destroyed, when the Sanidad had burned dwellings that had housed plague victims given the impossibility of disinfecting and fumigating these constructions. Offering compensation signaled a change in institutional practice; this had never been done, for instance, in the Alausí area. Such payment continued in 1929 when a new outbreak occurred in a neighboring area in the province.

Given the continuing importance of rats on railway cars in the spread of plague, Suárez also insisted that those who commercialized foodstuffs from Tungurahua and León provinces in the Guayaquil urban market modify the crates they used to ship their produce. His specific concern was that after the produce was unpacked in Guayaquil, the empty crates, often with fragments of cheese or butter or fruit still in them, waited in the railway warehouses to be shipped back to the central highlands. They attracted and harbored rats, which then traveled back to interior cities such as Ambato in the empty crates. The Sanidad developed two simple models of collapsible crates that could be built using the wood from the existing crates with the addition of some hardware. The medium merchants of Ambato protested bitterly about the expense and inconvenience involved, as did large landowners from the Guaytacama area such as the administrator of the Plaza-Lasso family's Hacienda La Avelina, but this was an issue on which Suárez (himself from Ambato) felt he was unable to compromise. Despite the unpopularity of this measure,[68] he saw it as necessary to the health and welfare of the nation. Indeed, the notion that public health defended a national interest that stood above private interests was actively being produced through these events and encounters.

Eradication and Reinfection

Once yellow fever had been eliminated from Guayaquil in 1919, the only obstacle to the city being declared a first-class clean port—significant for facilitating international trade—was the existence of plague. In 1929 anti-plague work further intensified in Ecuador and Peru with the arrival of the American Commission. Already plague was being brought under control in Guayaquil with the progress of the city's sanitation projects. Drs. Long and Eskey intensified anti-rat measures in Guayaquil, where an extensive poisoning campaign was in progress and traps were also used. In the port, public health inspector Luis Cajas developed an innovative system for delivering poison—at the time considered unique by the Pan American Sanitary Bureau[69]—in which wrapping paper was used to create small packets of poison mixed with flour and dried cod or cheese (which experience showed were the most effective of the various food stuffs tried). The first time an area was "covered" with poison packets, the less lethal poison barium carbonate was used, but once the human population was familiar with the poison packets, the more effective and less expensive arsenic was introduced into subsequent packets. Arsenic was also sufficiently slow acting that poisoned rats had time to crawl into hiding in concealed places removed from human contact before they died, precluding their fleas from finding human hosts. The variation in the packet contents helped to maintain effectiveness, as rats would not take the bait the second time an ingredient was used, leading to the establishment of a regular rotation of eight sets of ingredients in the packets.[70]

With new impetus to intensify urban anti-plague measures associated with the visit of Long and Eskey in 1929–1930, the disease was finally eliminated from Guayaquil, and to great jubilation the city formally qualified in 1930 as a class A-1 ("clean") port under the standards of the Pan American Sanitary Code.[71] From 1908 to 1930, the existence of plague in Guayaquil was seen as a threat to the highlands, particularly to Quito. Once plague was eliminated from Guayaquil in 1930, however, the perceived spatial threat changed substantially: it was now the highland region, especially Chimborazo province where plague had settled in, which was seen as a threat to both Guayaquil and the "international prestige" of Ecuador. A guiding assumption of anti-plague work up to 1930 was that if plague were eliminated from Guayaquil, it could be easily eradicated in the highlands as well. Experience proved this to be wrong.

At the same time as the American Commission was directing work in the port, they also began to investigate more systematically the causes of plague in the highlands, working with Ecuadorian officials such as Miño and the director of the Sanidad's newly created Technical Office, Ecuadorian bacteriologist Benjamín Wandemberg. Miño, Long, and Eskey also crossed the border from Loja into Peru in 1929 to meet with that country's public health officials to align regional efforts against plague. As Sanidad officials intensified their work in the highland provinces of

Loja and Chimborazo, they began to encounter new dynamics in the transmission of plague. The Loja provincial delegate had already pointed out in mid-1929 that, unlike urban areas affected by plague (Guayaquil and Ambato), his province faced multiple and simultaneous outbreaks in distant areas of the countryside.[72] In one clinical history that he reported in detail the next year because it was so illustrative of the local circumstances of plague transmission, the delegate showed how the family of a young unvaccinated Indigenous woman had received five cuyes from a family in a relatively distant Indigenous community and had eaten two, and then the remaining three cuyes had sickened and died. The young woman's fatal infection came soon thereafter.[73]

The 1929 measures to combat plague designed by Eskey reiterated quite clearly measures that were already being pursued in Ecuador, but the presence of the American Commission may have given them added credibility. For instance, for the epidemiological study of plague in Ecuador, Eskey recommended "the orderly collection of data concerning: the species of rats and their prevalence in diverse localities; the intensity of their infestation with fleas; the varieties of the latter; their correlation with the sex, age and species of rats; the variation in the number of fleas according to climatic conditions, the determination of plague epizooty, its exact diagnosis, and its intensity according to seasons."[74] This line of research was already ongoing in Ecuador under Suárez and his successor as director general, Dr. Alfonso Mosquera Narváez.[75] Long also drew on this prior work in preparing a concise memorandum about plague in Ecuador.[76] He highlights how plague transmission differed in the urban coast and the rural highlands. In Guayaquil, plague was transmitted by *cheopis* fleas who fed on infected rats. Therefore, it was necessary to trap rats, poison them, and alter architecture to make it rat-proof. Supplementary activities should include collecting and disposing of garbage, protecting foodstuffs, and identifying and isolating human cases. "With the elimination of plague in the lowlands," he asserts, "there are good reasons to assume that it will be easy to eradicate it in the highlands, because those areas will no longer be re-infected through their contact with the lowlands." In the highlands a different approach was needed, because neither the *cheopis* flea nor the rat was a primary transmitter of plague. Instead, Long suggests the following:

> There are persuasive reasons to believe that plague is extended from village to village, and sometimes even to towns, by human carriers—Indians—who carry infected fleas in their clothing, given their custom of attending wakes for those who have died of plague, where they become infested with fleas and where they themselves become infected and sicken some time

later after returning to their communities. Often the fleas that the Indians carry back with them then infect the guinea pigs that they keep in their huts, thus forming a reservoir of infection quite different from the rats that constitute that reservoir in the lowlands.

While Long was optimistic about the ease of eradicating plague in the highlands, doing so did not depend solely on scientific knowledge. The 1930s was a period of significant political and economic instability in Ecuador. Highland public health authorities repeatedly pleaded with the central government in the early 1930s for funds that would allow them to carry out the program set out by Long and Eskey to eliminate plague from Chimborazo in particular, with grave warnings about the risks to the port. As they feared, in 1935 Guayaquil was indeed reinfected with plague, despite the ongoing intensive rat catching and rat-proofing in the port city after 1930. In April 1935, a day laborer who worked unloading trains in the Durán rail terminus sickened with plague in a poor neighborhood of Guayaquil, Quinta Pareja; the origin of this case was traced back to Alausí. In August, another case was reported in Quinta Pareja, followed by more than one hundred additional cases in the city before the end of the year. It is a sign of how devastating the reinfection of Guayaquil was for the Sanidad's aspirations that director general Mosquera Narváez voluntarily offered to transfer the central office of the service back to Guayaquil to combat the disease more effectively, in an unusual relinquishment of authority that reduced him to a regional subdirector of the service under the new Guayaquil director general. It was only in 1939 that plague was considered "virtually eradicated" again in Guayaquil, after several years of infection. In 1940, Guayaquil was again declared a clean port.[77]

Ultimately, it is possible that the competition among rat species contributed to the elimination of plague in the port,[78] allowing for the reestablishment and maintenance of plague-free status even in moments of reduced government funding. Black rats (*Rattus rattus*) were introduced to the Americas in Columbus's first voyage, and there is evidence that they have inhabited Guayaquil since the 1540s (soon after the Spanish conquest of the Inca Empire). When plague arrived on ship rats in the early twentieth century, infection would have spread to local black rats that had not developed immunities, resulting in rapid deaths after which their fleas would have jumped off in search of other hosts, including human beings. No earlier than 1870, the more aggressive brown rat (*Rattus norvegicus*) had arrived in Guayaquil. Black rats are the preferred host of the *cheopis* flea and, as inside-dwelling rodents, also host more fleas than brown rats. The black rat also has smaller litters than the brown rat. In the end, it may be that the measures to reduce living quarters for black rats (climbers, rather than burrowers like the brown rats) combined with efforts to reduce urban waste—the food sources shared by brown and black rats—provided an advantage to the brown rat population. While black and brown rats can coexist if pressure on food resources is low, where such pressure does exist, the more prolific, omnivorous, and aggressive brown rat tends to outcompete the black rat. Geographer Daniel Gade reports that by the end of the twentieth century the brown rat had almost completely replaced the black rat in Guayaquil.

Plague ecology was different in Chimborazo, where other rodents and species of fleas were more commonly the transmitters of plague. The tone of the campaigns in Chimborazo became increasingly harsh following the elimination of plague from Guayaquil, and even more so after the reinfection of the port. Indigenous culture and hygiene began to be identified explicitly as the cause of the continued existence of plague in Ecuador. A number of Indigenous practices were highlighted, such as human cohabitation with cuyes. As Long had suggested, the transmission of plague from Indigenous village to village was judged to be due to Indigenous behavior at *velorios* (wakes) following the death of a community member. Often a velorio took place in the same hut in which the victim had lived, where "the participants drink large quantities of *chicha* [corn beer], become intoxicated, and fall asleep on the floor of the *choza*. As this harbors infected fleas, the Indians are infected or carry back to their dwellings infected fleas, leading to a new outbreak of the disease."[79] The American Commission had recommended the construction of funeral huts so that wakes were not held in the locations where people died of plague. Indigenous peasants also tended to redistribute the clothing of the dead rather than burn it as public health authorities insisted. Finally, in cases of *viruela pestosa*, anyone who touched a victim's cadaver could release the infected pus. During velorios, Indigenous people caressed and washed the cadavers of plague victims.

In addition to customs surrounding death, other Indigenous practices were also identified as dangerous. A rare form of plague that appeared in Indigenous areas was *angina pestosa*, characterized by violent swelling of the throat; this was attributed to "the Indians' custom of killing fleas with their teeth when they are found on their person or clothing." Another practice was to eat animals that had died, whether cuyes or wild rabbits; if they had died of plague, infection of humans was possible. Altogether, it was thought that only the cold climate and high altitudes of the zones where Indigenous communities were located prevented plague from being even more virulent. In 1940, the director of the Ecuadorian anti-plague office (a formal section by then in the Sanidad's Guayaquil central office) was struck by the fact that "the rate of morbidity in the different outbreaks is relatively low, despite the terrible hygienic conditions in which the Indians live, and their repugnant customs of consuming dead animals they encounter and chewing ticks and fleas, favorable conditions for an outbreak of great proportions, without this having happened except in very few cases."[80] He struggled to understand why infection rates were not higher, given his assessment of Indigenous customs.

From August 1942 to July 1943, an intensive campaign was carried out in Chimborazo, with $50,000 in funding from the Institute for Inter-American Affairs, a new US agency that was increasingly involved in funding health initiatives in Ecuador in the Second World War era (for instance, participating in the construction of the first Centro de Salud in Quito adjacent to the colonial-era Hospital San Juan de Dios and supporting the establishment of a new professional nursing school annexed to the Universidad Central[81]). In this rural anti-plague campaign, emphasis was placed on the elimination of fleas. By the 1940s it had been determined that plague-infected fleas could survive for months in a dormant state and then reappear with a favorable change in climatic conditions, explaining why there could be a resurgence of plague without being preceded by epizootics in rodents.[82] In the Chimborazo campaign, rodent caves and nests were destroyed by means of use of cyanide gas for nests in the walls and roofs of chozas and flame throwers for outside work in ravines.

The extermination of rodents continued to be of key importance. As the director of the Ecuadorian anti-plague campaign explains in 1943, "the extermination of guinea pigs has been one of the measures to which we have dedicated preferential attention, even though it has brought us the greatest difficulties and bother given the affection that the population has for these little creatures; a population that due to its ignorance has posed the most absurd resistance to the extermination of these rodents, provoking serious conflicts. Nonetheless the number of guinea pigs exterminated this year is quite considerable and currently there are many sectors in which it is difficult to find any at all."[83] This was considered especially important because at times plague appeared in widely distant areas simultaneously, which was thought to be due to the active exchange of cuyes among members of different Indigenous communities (as the 1929 Loja case suggested), an Andean custom with deep roots.[84] The campaign also aimed to change the way Indigenous people lived in more general terms, as is made clear by the leader of the anti-plague office:

> The work of hygiene in general in the countryside has been carried out despite the difficulties posed by a population completely lacking in the most elemental norms of hygiene, and that lives in the most complete filth and the most horrifying promiscuity with all kinds of animals. In spite of these adverse conditions, I think that we have achieved an improvement in hygiene, but given the tendencies of the Indigenous population, I doubt very much that these good customs will be conserved when we cannot continue exercising the strict monitoring we have applied during the current year, during which we have carried out 189,048 domestic inspections.[85]

With this intensive work, he was proud to report that while in 1939 there were eighty-two cases of plague in Chimborazo, in 1940 there were forty cases, in 1941 thirty-nine cases, in 1942 there was only one, and in the first half of 1943 there were no *reported* cases. It is possible, of course, that a hardening of the methods used among the Indigenous population—clearly returning to an emphasis on containment over care—might itself have contributed to hiding cases, undermining the aims of the campaign. Indeed, as late as 1998 there was an isolated outbreak of plague in the Indigenous community of Nisag in the Alausí canton, where the photo presented in this book's Introduction had been taken some seven decades earlier.

The immediate catalyst for the establishment of Ecuador's Sanidad service, plague continued to play an important role in the changing structure of the agency through the 1930s, when the service's main office was moved back to Guayaquil following the port's 1935 reinfection. The history of plague and anti-plague measures in Ecuador shows an increasing specificity in how the disease was understood and also illustrates well some of the early financial and institutional constraints faced by public health reformers. This history also shows changing notions of the dangers posed by plague that reflected not only scientific knowledge but also social, ethnic, and regional relations, as the balance between containment and care continued to shift (with implications for how the population experienced and responded to public health projects).

In thinking about state formation and state effects in light of Ecuador's plague experience, the correspondence among leaders of the Sanidad shows that they did not see the public health service as coterminous with the government. Instead, they clearly distinguished themselves, as technical experts, from the government, made up of elected politicians. In doing so, they were developing their own identity as nonpolitical state actors. After the 1925 Revolución Juliana, when a group of social reformers with a nationalist bent came to power, this took a more robust form, which can be seen most clearly in the Guaytacama plague campaign. The Sanidad was not only fighting plague, relatively successfully, in that campaign (with no further cases in the area after June 1926) but also developing an image of the state as standing apart from and above society—and able to intervene in it. This was manifested in such actions as the ability to intervene in conflicts and procure, for instance, equally the jailing of would-be rapists and the freeing from jail of the leaders of Indigenous uprisings. It was manifested even more in relation to large landowners of the zone when, despite their financial contributions toward the plague campaign and seeming alignment with the project, the Sanidad leadership was unwilling to compromise on the requirement that they modify their packing crates. Standing strong against landowner complaints in the name of the national interest was especially symbolic in this specific region.[86] Just a decade earlier, the very same large landowners who supported the plague campaign had used their connections with elected politicians to push through legislation that promoted their own economic interests as the general interest, in the form of the 1918 Law of Agricultural Development (which was drafted by Gangotena Jijón's Sociedad Nacional de Agricultura and presented to the minister of agriculture, who sent it on to congress).[87] And finally, the Sanidad did not hesitate to distinguish itself from more political appointees of the government during the Guaytacama outbreaks by requesting that executive appointees at all levels (provincial governor, canton-level political administrator, and parish-level political lieutenant) be fined for their active or passive undermining of public health orders.

Striking in this period was the lack of pathologization of Indigenous behavior. Instead, public health officials were engaged in the development of more general norms of appropriate and healthy behavior among all social classes, who had a role to play that was seen as complementary to the work of the state in this area. However, once plague was eliminated from Guayaquil, increasing frustration was shown with the Indigenous populations and rural Andean areas where plague had found a new reservoir, altering the perceived ethnicity of plague and indicating a new "geography of blame" (to use Paul Farmer's term).[88] The reinfection of Guayaquil seemed to mark a further hardening of the structure of blame and the identification of certain Indigenous practices as repugnant. This may have also been linked to the concentration of anti-plague work in the Guayaquil central office of the Sanidad after 1935, where public health officials might have had less familiarity with Andean Indigenous culture. While undoubtedly in some cases familiarity bred contempt of Indigenous culture, in other cases it encouraged more paternalistic understandings. Suárez, for instance, grew up in Ambato and the surrounding countryside. His writings on Indigenous life in the 1930s were undoubtedly ideologically tinged,[89] but they lacked the harshness of the passages cited above.[90] By the early 1940s, the service seemed to rely more on technical fixes via the use of cyanide gas and flame throwers (and, soon thereafter, DDT) than on building trust with Indigenous communities.[91] In his analysis of evolving notions of the rat's role in plague in colonial India, anthropologist Nicholas Evans highlights how, as technical knowledge was gained, public health approaches to plague retreated from more complex multifactorial explanations to singular ones based on germ theory, in ways that centered blame on colonized people.[92] Ironically, in Ecuador, the negative comments about Indigenous peasants' backwardness came at a time when Indigenous communities were forging links with each other, with urban workers, and with political parties,[93] one product of which was the 1944 establishment of the Federación Ecuatoriana de Indios (FEI). Indeed, the denigration and dehumanizing language used about them suggests backlash against their emergence as political actors on a broader stage. Just as the balance between care and containment did not move in a single direction, so too state practices toward and rhetoric about the Indigenous population exhibited both advances and retreats.

In his discussion of the work of governing, John Clarke argues that "governments have to perform being governments for a range of audiences, located in different settings and formed in different relationships, demonstrating their competence and capacity."[94] Public health officials did seem to have an awareness of audience, which does not mean these performances were empty show. While state practices were rooted in a matrix of social and political relations, this chapter suggests how Sanidad leaders tried to position themselves as above social conflicts, generating in the process notions of a national interest that was above partisan politics and narrower private interests. It points, too, to the difficulties of establishing personnel networks that would allow the service to reach into new spaces, demonstrating and indeed generating their capacity. We turn to a closer consideration of these and related problems in the next chapter.

Chapter 2

Forging Public Health as State Idea and State System

> The Sanidad service is a true administrative function that the State has reason to exercise with increasing activity and enthusiasm, in order to achieve the result of a healthy and robust, and therefore vigorous and enterprising, population. Today no civilized people exists that does not consider its progress to depend, in large part, on perfecting its public health service.
>
> **—José María Ayora, Minister of the Interior, 1912**

Ecuador's encounter with plague partly depended on refining scientific knowledge of the disease ecology of Ecuadorian plague, a process to which Ecuadorian public health physicians and workers contributed. However, those experiences also revealed that public health projects depend on much more than the progress of medical research. The development of networks of personnel, funding levels, and interpersonal relations within and between institutions and with the public also had a significant impact on what kinds of activities were possible. In this chapter we delve into factors of this kind, related to the incremental assembling of public health as a state system, which influenced the contours of possibilities, pressures, and constraints on public health practices. All of that, however, depends on a logically prior question: Just how and when did the notion emerge that public health was a legitimate and necessary area of government activity?

This chapter takes seriously Philip Abrams's suggestion that we distinguish the state system and the state idea, recognize their specific features in particular contexts, and explore how they relate to each other.[1] It is also inspired by Andrew Abbott's discussion of the system of professions—in which he argues that practitioners exist within a kind of ecosystem where they engage and compete with each other for space[2]—here, extending his approach by situating the Sanidad as a state agency in a broader ecosystem of institutions and actors. The chapter begins with an exploration of the broad outlines of an emerging state idea in which public health came to be seen as an appropriate arena for administrative activity. That idea was developed alongside and in contrast to existing notions about "beneficencia" as an organized expression of charitable social welfare activity. Then it turns to how the state system of public health began to be cobbled together unevenly across the national territory, with a growing infrastructure of offices and personnel who needed internally to develop means of coordinating with each other and externally to manage and negotiate relations with actors such as municipal governments, social welfare institutions, and private physicians, among others. The period 1925–1926 was a watershed moment when these awkward and uneven iterative growths were reorganized into a coherent system. Or, at least, that was the deepening state idea of how public health operated, despite some evidence to the contrary in everyday practice.

The Rise of the Idea of Public Health in Ecuador

The fact that when bubonic plague arrived in Ecuador in 1908 there was no national institution charged with overseeing and intervening in public health matters suggests that it is not self-evident that health issues should be considered of either national scope or state concern. What position did health in general hold in notions of public administration, then, at the turn of the twentieth century, and how did the role of public health in particular emerge as an area of legitimate government concern and activity? Subsequent chapters explore further how this notion was activated and strengthened through a variety of encounters, but first, the broad framing of health issues as a justifiable area of state activity at the national level is traced here in the annual reports of the minister of the interior, who oversaw a wide range of portfolios as one of only four or five cabinet ministers at the turn of the century. While the various sections within the ministries were periodically reorganized and reallocated, the ministries generally included ones dedicated to interior matters (Ministerio de lo Interior), foreign relations (Relaciones Exteriores), justice (Justicia), finance (Hacienda, or sometimes Hacienda y Crédito Público), and education (Instrucción Pública). The titles of their reports suggest the broad scope of these ministries: "Ministro de lo Interior, Municipalidades, Policía, Obras Públicas, etc.," with much falling under the "etc."[3] These annual reports were carefully constructed public documents summarizing, for congress or sometimes for "the nation," government activity over the previous year situated in its social and political context.

As the new government fought to consolidate its rule after the 1895 Liberal Revolution and struggled with the civil unrest associated with the secularization projects that would eventually produce the separation of church and state, health-related language was used metaphorically to comment on the effects of clerical actions on society in general and especially on the poor population. Thus in 1897 the minister of the interior muses in his annual report: "It is good that there is religion in society, because to some extent it is necessary for its proper functioning; but not imposed on us as it has been, like a crippling burden weighing down the strongest population: with a convent on every corner and in every house, people sweat drops of blood to be able to afford the so-called holy sacraments that are administered to them like high-priced drugs, supposedly for their health, when in truth they are being administered the slow and agonizing death that is called destitution, while the priests are awash in luxury and comfort."[4] Moving beyond metaphor, for the first time since the 1895 revolution, health issues were discussed explicitly in the 1902 report of the minister, in a brief, newly incorporated section on "Hygiene" in the annual report. The minister argues there that physical health is linked to the circulation of new ideas and therefore to social progress, evoking other public discussions about awakening the country from lethargy through reducing the influence of the Catholic Church, reforming education, and building infrastructure.[5] He points out that "malnourished peoples, consuming toxic food articles, lodged in narrow rooms without sufficient air circulation, will never march at the forefront of civilization. But with good nutrition and pure air; discouraging the consumption of alcohol and tobacco; preventing the thousand sophistications that industry introduces each day into articles of primary necessity, our people could have rich and well-oxygenated blood that, on arriving in the brain, could awaken ideas and communicate vigor and strength to the muscles."[6] To further these goals, he proposes the creation of numerous new offices and agencies to operationalize these ideas: a separate section of Higiene and Sanidad within the Ministry of the Interior; a Consejo Supremo de Sanidad e Higiene; Juntas de Higiene Provincial; a Junta de Sanidad in Quito; Institutos de Higiene in both Quito and Guayaquil; and a reorganization of the Junta de Sanidad de Guayaquil (which had been established in 1899). Few of these recommendations were acted upon in the short term.[7]

Already the following year this language seemed antiquated, with more specific health threats looming on the horizon that made it apparent that new organizational structures and practices might indeed be required. However, ongoing challenges involved in the separation of church and state were still in the foreground. The minister reports in 1903 on such issues:

> As if the attitude assumed by the Ecuadorian Episcopate and the conservative press against the Law of Civil Marriage—an attitude that produced deep unease in the spirits of the majority—had not been enough to create a state of public anguish . . . ; as if last year's disasters that reduced to ashes flourishing settlements [likely the July 1902 fire that devastated Guayaquil], were not enough to fill hearts with despair; as if the yellow fever epidemic that caused so many victims in Guayaquil was not sufficient motive for fear and despondency; the announcement of a new scourge, and the very nearness of it, was the final drop that caused an overflow of profound alarm in the country. The bubonic plague—ominous traveler that, emerging from the Indostanic regions, carries desolation everywhere without respect to climates or latitudes—has appeared in the Peruvian ports of Callao and Pisco.[8]

Thus the list of disasters disheartening Ecuadorians at the time included conservative opposition to secularization, massive fires, and two specific deadly diseases. However, it was the first of these—struggles with conservatives and the Catholic Church over the separation of church and state, coupled with internecine struggles among liberals over political succession—that dominated the report of the minister over the following five years.

Even so, a separate section on "Beneficencia" began to be included regularly in the annual reports of the minister of the interior, covering a range of social welfare issues. While social welfare and public health were on the verge of being distinguished from each other, in the 1908 report, the section on beneficencia largely outlined activities that soon would come to be defined as sanidad—namely, the measures taken against the bubonic plague outbreak in the port. The minister highlighted the contribution of US physicians to the laboratory identification of plague in Guayaquil; the creation of a Comisión Especial de Saneamiento by executive decree on March 24, 1908; the subsequent establishment again by executive decree of a Junta Superior de Higiene y Sanidad in both Quito and Cuenca, with jurisdiction respectively in the north-central highland provinces and the southern highland provinces; and the creation of a Comisión Especial de Higiene y Saneamiento del Ferrocarril with jurisdiction between the Durán rail terminus and Alausí composed of three physicians appointed by the minister. Importantly, the minister concluded with the recommendation that the sanitation of Guayaquil be declared a national project (*obra nacional*)—in other words, not just one of local interest or sustained by local funding—and that Congress vote sufficient earmarked funds from the national budget to ensure this project could be carried out.[9]

In 1908 both beneficencia and sanidad experienced significant new forms of institutionalization, which began to distinguish more clearly between these spheres of activity. In early November 1908 the Ley de Sanidad (Law of Public Health), discussed further below, established the public health service. A couple of weeks earlier, a new Ley de Beneficencia, in turn, had authorized the formal expropriation of the property of foreign religious orders, whose proceeds were henceforth dedicated to social welfare programs administered by regional Juntas de Beneficencia (with a portion of these funds also used to support the expenses of the religious orders). This built on the 1904 Ley de Cultos that had required religious orders to submit annual budgets outlining their essential operating expenses for approval by the government, with any excess income from their rural estates being channeled to support projects as determined by the government.[10] While beneficencia programs had been managed by the Catholic Church in the colonial period,[11] following the 1895 Liberal Revolution the laws outlined here helped the state to establish its own role and authority over social welfare institutions as well as, more generally, over the Catholic Church, joining laws promoting civil marriage, civil registry, and changes in the public education system that advanced liberal projects to secularize society.[12]

Given that these changes to beneficencia activities were the result of ongoing negotiations in specific historical and social contexts, it is worth pausing to note that there was a marked regional difference in the way that beneficencia services were organized and funded in Ecuador. For historical reasons related in part to the spatial distribution of the population, the vast majority of the rural and urban real estate of religious orders was located in the highlands rather than in the coastal region, which had been more sparsely populated during the colonial period. When the liberal government expropriated the real estate of religious orders in the first decade of the twentieth century and dedicated the rental fees paid by leaseholders to social welfare and other development projects in the region in which properties were located, this generated greater resources for the north-central highlands (characterized by larger estates and more fertile soils) than for the southern highlands, and more in both cases than for the coast due to the smaller number of religious properties in the latter.

Perhaps partly due to the relatively weaker presence of Catholic institutions in the coastal region, social welfare in Guayaquil had been organized since 1888 by the Junta de Beneficencia de Guayaquil (JBG),[13] established by the municipality for the purpose of "creating a system of organized charity." The previous year, at the request specifically of the Guayaquil municipal government, Congress had authorized municipalities in general to delegate their responsibility to administer hospitals and welfare institutions to autonomous juntas.[14] In its early years the JBG operated with some municipal funding and occasional contributions by the national government. Increasingly, however, JBG programs were supported by funds generated by the Junta's investments. For instance, in 1896, the JBG purchased the 3,600-hectare agricultural estate La Atarazana using 60,000 sucres that had been bequeathed to the Junta. This estate was about ten times the size of Guayaquil's urban area at the time; the income generated from leasing this land was considerable.[15] The JBG also had other income-generating activities, such as their popular lottery which enjoyed a national monopoly.[16] The 1908 Ley de Beneficencia that established regional Juntas in Quito and Cuenca left the existing Guayaquil Junta intact, specifying that "the Junta de Beneficencia Municipal de Guayaquil will continue in the form in which it is currently organized, and with absolute independence of this Law."[17]

Before the 1908 law, an 1896 presidential decree by Eloy Alfaro established a Junta de Beneficencia in Quito, composed of "35 honorable property owners," mirroring the size of the Guayaquil Junta. One difficulty in following the Guayaquil model, however, was that in more conservative Quito many such notables were initially opposed to the liberal government: as the minister's report in 1899 confirmed, this Junta had still not been fully established three years later due to ongoing political instability.[18] In 1901 there was another attempt to constitute this Junta in Quito. The 1908 law regularized considerably Beneficencia activities in the highlands by providing a more stable set of resources on which they could draw and a clearer structure to administer them.[19] In the minister's 1909 report, indeed, the Beneficencia section dealt primarily with the establishment of the regional Juntas and their budgeting process. The 1908 law also established a more modest size for the Juntas in Quito and Cuenca, each with two ex officio members (the provincial governor and the municipal council president of Quito or Cuenca) and three additional board members (*vocales*).

Around the same time, a national Ley de Sanidad was also passed. In the discussion of this legislation, President Alfaro's address to Congress regarding the urgent need to establish a national Sanidad service summed up the profound and wide-ranging importance of public health as well as its differential effects. "Modern international law requires that ports open to international commerce should be free from such diseases as plague, yellow fever, cholera, and smallpox; this is only right, inasmuch as the most important attribute of government is to protect the lives of its citizens. The propagation of such terrible diseases not only decimates our cities and retards their progress, but also causes the isolation of the nation so infested, and consequently, the ruin of its commerce and industries; it causes immense financial loss to the better classes and suffering and destitution among the poor."[20]

In 1909, for the first time "Sanidad" was separated out from Beneficencia in the annual report of the minister of the interior, following the establishment of the Servicio de Sanidad the previous November. The Sanidad section focused on disease prevention and organizational matters. One indication that the Servicio de Sanidad was a national state institution, and no longer just a municipal one, was that Congress was charged with naming its director. However, because the 1908 Congress had run out of time before appointing a director of Sanidad, the Council of State (Consejo de Estado) named US physician Bolívar Lloyd as interim director so that the work of this agency could proceed, including formulating appropriate regulations (Lloyd was replaced within a few months by Ecuadorian physician Luis Felipe Cornejo Gómez). The minister also reported that over the previous year, he had urged the provincial governors to continue putting into practice any measures ordered by his office regarding the sanitation of population centers; subdirectors of Sanidad had been appointed in various provinces; and the 1908 Ley de Sanidad required municipalities to include funds in their budgets for public health projects in their respective cantons.[21]

In extended coverage in the minister's 1910 annual report, the emerging fields of beneficencia and sanidad were more clearly defined, in ways that continued to characterize these areas of activity until the 1926 reconceptualization of the Beneficencia agency as Asistencia Pública (shifting emphasis from charity toward entitlement to public assistance or services). In 1910, the Beneficencia's activities were conceived in terms of the field's historical roots in charity. The two faces of beneficencia activities were thus described as "helping the poor who cannot work [and] impeding poverty. For the first, Hospitals, Orphanages, Asylums, etc. have been created; for the second, the State has a duty to ensure the establishment of Cajas de Ahorro, Montes de Piedad, Casas de Préstamo, etc." The minister went on to remark that "all of the sources of human misery find their remedy in the altruistic action of the Juntas: the orphan and the aged have their shelter, the leper and the madman have their refuge, and the ill recover their health in the hospital." The role of the ministry was simply to encourage and approve the activities of the "distinguished citizens" who comprised these institutions.[22] In other words, while the state had an oversight role, beneficencia was largely presented as a private sphere of activity. Indeed, the JBG was fiercely protective of its autonomy—successfully so, as it was not required to adapt its activities to the new 1908 national law governing Beneficencia programs. While pursuing their activities under municipal auspices, the members of the Junta were private citizens rather than municipal employees, and general statements repeatedly alluded to the energetic private philanthropic thrust of the Junta's activities. In the highlands, too, the members of the Juntas de Beneficencia were private citizens, not state employees, although the funding for their activities was generated more directly by state actions (via its expropriation of the real estate of religious orders).[23]

Discussion of Sanidad activities came later in the minister's 1910 report—not only no longer merged with Beneficencia but separated from it by several other sections of the report—and expresses a markedly more muscular vision of state responsibility for national health and well-being:

> From the principle that the State is an organic being, very important consequences have been deduced for the political life of peoples—its immediate corollary being the duty it has to preserve the human personality, individually and collectively considered. If, then, man is the primary element in the political organization of nations, it is unquestionable that his preservation is one of its primordial goals. The duty that the Government has to attend to the health and well-being of its associates translates into the administrative function of *public health* [emphasis in the original]. It is understandable that concern for the health of man is due to the powerful sense of self-preservation; even more when the dangers that threaten a people are of great transcendence, whether due to the easy propagation of contagious diseases or the impossibility of the individual alone to confront epidemics, thus the social collectivity has an interest in eliminating the germs of death that attack it. But to channel individual actions, conveniently regulating them, the immediate and decisive cooperation of the Public Power ["Poder Público," or the state] is needed and for these reasons this labor acquires the character of an administrative function and the duties it has are proportionate to the gravity of the dangers threatening the population.[24]

The minister further pointed out that public health was a function specifically of *modern* states, a sign of the times in which the development of medical and physical sciences made it possible to establish public health as a social duty of human collectivities. He then went on to outline the negative and positive dimensions of public health work—namely, efforts on the one hand to eliminate health risks through medical and other interventions and on the other to improve sanitation conditions as preventive measures. These actions would be carried out by the two elements that made up the service—"administrative action," the efforts of the Public Power to preserve and promote health, and the "technical element," composed of the specialized scientific knowledge of the personnel charged with responsibility for public health. In sum, sanidad was first justified as an area of state responsibility for the good of the collectivity and then was conceived as a technical activity that relied on specialized knowledge, backed up by administrative power. This made it very different, then, from beneficencia, where even the curative side of medical activities was still linked to the historic role of the hospital as a refuge or shelter for the socially marginalized—and, for the ill, perhaps more a place to die than a place to recuperate. The emphasis on public health's novel character based on the advances of modern science further distinguished it from beneficencia.

Ministerial reports persisted in this vein in subsequent years, emphasizing that society should be grateful for the assiduous, selfless, and philanthropic efforts of the Juntas de Beneficencia. Public health, however, continued in 1912 to be justified in strong terms as an area of direct state activity. Continuing the comments provided in the epigraph to this chapter, the minister asked: "What could be more natural than the vital goal of countering, by all means possible, the destructive effects of those diseases which decimate in little time the populations they invade, and the attempt to prevent or remedy—according to the situation—such ills by the measures that scientific advance has achieved in the areas of hygiene, sanitation, and curation. The reduction in the mortality caused by infecto-contagious diseases is a problem that is related fundamentally to social progress, for the very simple reason that good health is the sine qua non foundation of all intellectual, moral and material progress."[25] The much newer area of public health evidently required more active justification than beneficencia, and the state's role in it, too, was quite different. Public health was not primarily about individual suffering, but rather it elevated the social collectivity above the individual, focusing on the needs of the larger population in ways that allowed for and supported new forms of monitoring of and intervention into people's lives. At the same time, the emphasis on the "technical element" in public health work positioned Sanidad workers as nonpolitical. As the minister sums up the state's role in public health in his 1914 report, "The administration's responsibility to facilitate all of the conditions necessary for uninhibited social improvement is undeniable; and it is also its duty to maintain the right to life, that is, to protect Sanidad and hygiene, removing all that may damage health and supporting all that may favor it. Individual action is not sufficient to overcome the causes that produce perturbations to our collective organism, weakening it, ruining it, and destroying it."[26]

The rapid evolution in how health issues were framed as a matter of state concern in just a dozen years is striking: while public health was still generally linked to notions of social progress, it was framed both in more specifically medical terms and as an appropriate and necessary area of state intervention. This reflects changing political dynamics as the liberal government program moved on from its early radical phase focused on secularization to begin to expand the scope of its activities. It also reflects new threats to the nation posed by deadly diseases like plague. The ministerial and presidential statements above suggest that the scale of the threat informed the argument that a national (indeed, a national *state*) response was needed: due not only to the degree of danger but also as a result of the plague's potential to spread across and around the national territory. While individuals were threatened by disease, society—"the social collectivity," or "our collective organism"—was also threatened, and it was in its name that the state acted. However, the means by which state actors could develop the capacity to do so were neither obvious nor easy.

Assembling the State System of Public Health

As we have seen, there were some ambitious ideas expressed by government leaders in the first decade of the twentieth century about how the Ecuadorian state should intervene to protect the broader social interest through public health measures. Any attempt to do so, however, required not just an appropriate state idea but also a compatible state system that could convert statements of principle into practices. As outlined above, in Guayaquil there was both the semiprivate-municipal Junta de Beneficencia established in 1888 and, from 1899, the municipal Junta Superior de Sanidad Marítima y Urbana (or Board of Health) as well. The creation of the Servicio de Sanidad with funding from the national budget was a different matter—it was not a local council of municipal and port officials but a national government service. The regulations framed by the director of the service were legally binding on residents and thus, in the early years, had to be reviewed by a commission consisting of the deans of both the faculties of medicine and law and one other member of each of these faculties at the Universidad de Guayaquil, with the university rector presiding over the commission. By this means, a state university was initially in a supervisory role over the state public health service (chapter 5 outlines some changes to the relations between universities and the Sanidad in subsequent decades).

The 1908 Ley de Sanidad specified that the personnel of the service should be physicians to the extent possible, led in Guayaquil by the director and two physician assistants, and with a subdirector and two assistants "for each city or town where their services were needed."[27] The director and two assistants in Guayaquil had salaries assigned in the Ley de Sanidad, while the costs of public health services in other locations were to be covered by the local municipal governments. Once the Ley de Sanidad took effect, the existing Board of Health in Guayaquil and the Comisión Especial would be disbanded and their equipment, supplies, offices, and funds transferred to the Sanidad.

The initial funding for this national service reconfigured a budget of 240,000 sucres (20,000 per month) approved by the national government for the sanitation of Guayaquil, which would be used to cover the service's salaries, purchase of materials, costs of maintaining quarantine facilities, and the like. Additional extraordinary funds could be approved by the national president in the case of disease outbreaks elsewhere. Guayaquil clearly had a unique position in the national territory when it came to public health concerns. Its concentrated urban population and vulnerability to tropical disease outbreaks gave it a reputation as the pesthole of the Pacific.[28] Given its central role as the country's main port, as we have seen health conditions there could have broad ramifications for the national economy if international trade was interrupted as a result. And the fact that the import-export taxes assessed at the Guayaquil customs house made a significant contribution to the national budget in the first place may well have also been a consideration in (re)directing these funds to Guayaquil. The substantial nature of the financial resources placed under the control of the director general of Sanidad was underlined by the detailed provisions in the body of the law about the financial guarantees that the director must offer and the penalties he would suffer for any misuse of these funds (provisions that were covered exhaustively in the law's longest article). Unlike Guayaquil, in other locations where public health work needed to be undertaken, local municipal governments were expected to dedicate funds to these projects and were permitted to establish new taxes in order to do so, as it was widely recognized that the existing resources of municipalities were not sufficient to provide expanded services. While new responsibilities were placed on municipalities, they may have welcomed the permission to establish new taxes and generally to engage in local fundraising.

While the Sanidad was a national institution in terms of receiving funding from the national government, for the first six years of its operation, only the city of Guayaquil had permanently stationed staff charged with confronting public health issues. When other towns or cities in Ecuador experienced disease outbreaks, a traveling commission might be sent from the Guayaquil headquarters to carry out eradication campaigns in affected areas, usually paid for by locally generated municipal revenues, sometimes in combination with some national funding if the risk were sufficiently high (typically using extraordinary rather than budgeted funds). There were attempts to create subdirector positions for the national service in other locations, but lack of funding did not allow them to consolidate their operations. In 1908 in Quito there was an inspector of hygiene who was also called the subdirector of Sanidad—lawyer Francisco Andrade Marín—working out of the Oficina de Higiene Municipal funded and overseen by the city's municipal government. By 1910 there was a separate municipal director of the Oficina de Higiene Municipal—by then a physician, Dr. Francisco Martínez Serrano—as well as a subdirector of Sanidad for Pichincha province, Dr. Angel Sáenz. However, the Quito municipality only funded Sáenz's salary while providing no other supplies or staff, leading Sáenz himself to recommend that either there be appropriate funding for the office's activities or it be disbanded. As the minister reports, reflecting on Sáenz's comments, it was shameful that a simple lack of resources prevented such important work. In an appropriately biological metaphor, he argues more generally that "it is necessary to bring to life the aforementioned Subdirectorates, which, in their current form, are nothing more than cadavers, due to the lack of funds." Even though the Ley de Sanidad required municipalities to dedicate necessary funds to public health, "it is notorious that the municipal councils, which barely have enough for the most strictly urgent of their obligations, are never in a situation to be able to attend to any new responsibilities established by the Ley de Sanidad, without the generation of additional sources of income."[29] In October 1912, Sáenz's position was indeed eliminated, given lack of funds to continue sustaining the precarious subdirectorate.[30]

Early on there were also subdirectors of Sanidad appointed temporarily in the coastal provinces Manabí and Los Ríos, but again without stable funding and status. In the two Manabí port towns of Bahía and Manta, subdirectors were appointed in January 1912 and February 1913. There was also a subdirectorate of Sanidad established in highland Chimborazo province with the 1913 arrival of plague in Alausí. Dr. Carlos Miño traveled from Alausí, where he was leading the anti-plague campaign, to provincial capital Riobamba to organize the personnel and budget of the subdirectorate, and Dr. Juan Esteves took up the subdirector position on April 19, 1913. Over the following months Esteves oversaw a physician assistant, office staff, fumigators, disinfection squads, two rat catchers, two ten-man squads for general sanitation, and a group of vaccinators for both urban and rural areas. This staff numbered forty-two in the 1913 annual report for the Sanidad service. Nonetheless, the Chimborazo subdirectorate was more fleeting than it seemed, and the entire office was eliminated in months when plague declined and then reestablished when the disease reappeared.

Elsewhere, too, subdirectorates of Sanidad were precarious. In January 1915, the Los Ríos subdirectorate located in provincial capital Babahoyo was eliminated because the municipality redirected the funds for Sanidad work to the construction of a jail. Similarly, in June 1915 the municipal council of Bahía in Manabí eliminated the Sanidad service because the budgeted funds had been exhausted. Meanwhile in Manta in 1915 a physician was serving as the Sanidad delegate *ad honorem* (on an unpaid basis) until something better could be devised. In mid-1915 it was considered urgent to reestablish the Riobamba subdirectorate, which had been suspended temporarily. Sanidad director general León Becerra also thought it imperative to create subdirectorates in Machala and Esmeraldas (on the southern and northern coast, respectively) as "advanced sentinels protecting the country's borders against exotic pestilential diseases, such as cholera, which is a constant threat along the Pacific coast."[31] Like biological metaphors, military metaphors were also common in describing public health work.

Just as commissions might be sent out from Guayaquil to smaller cities or towns, five years after the establishment of the Sanidad service in Guayaquil in August 1913 a commission was sent to Quito to confer on infectious disease control measures there. The commission leader, Dr. Miño, initially was in the capital as a delegate of the Guayaquil directorate from August through December, until his position was converted to a permanent one as Quito subdirector of the national service effective January 1914. As the director general explains, "The threat that plague would invade the capital and the urgency of taking energetic and well-directed hygienic measures were motive for the reestablishment of the subdirectorate of Sanidad in Quito."[32] Henceforth, from 1914 the capital and the port both had permanently stationed public health staff, although for the ensuing dozen years they were still the only two Ecuadorian cities that did.[33] Miño's appointment had a much more stable status than other more ephemeral subdirectors, as the director general confirms in his 1915 annual report: "Only the subdirectorate in Quito functions with regularity and carries out important work with practical results, both due to the competence of its director and to the unusual circumstance that it is assigned funds through the national budget; the subdirectorates in other locations cannot subsist, indeed they don't really exist, due to the lack of their own funds, as they are subject to the resources and whims of the municipalities."[34] Nonetheless, when the Quito subdirectorate was first established it was unable to collect its monthly funding for January 1914 from the national government until June that year.[35]

Undoubtedly the levels of funding available to establish and extend public health activities exerted significant constraints on what was possible. In his 1915 report, Becerra highlights the many inadequacies of the service that "generally result from the deficient funding provided, which could easily be remedied if the Congress would decentralize completely these funds so that they would not be exposed to the vagaries and contingencies of politics which affect public institutions such as the Sanidad when they do not enjoy economic autonomy."[36] Becerra's frustration was likely fueled by the fact that, a few months earlier, the service's monthly funding had been reduced by half, from 20,000 sucres to 10,000 sucres for the entire service. In 1915–1916, as the export crisis associated with the First World War deepened, the monthly funding that had initially been promised for the operations of the Quito subdirectorate was reduced from 10,000 sucres to 2,000 sucres, and in some months only 700 sucres were actually paid out by the treasury.[37] In May 1916, some staff positions in the Quito office were eliminated due to the lack of resources for salaries. The subdirectorate managed to cobble together some funds to pay for essential expenses by taking over direct collection of public health fees rather than farming them out.[38] In Guayaquil, Becerra's frequent use throughout 1916 of his own personal stationery to communicate business of the Sanidad is another indication of the straitened economic circumstances of the service.

Funding was indeed a chronic problem, even in Quito and Guayaquil which were allocated monies through the national budget (and where municipal resources might also generally be greater than in other cities or towns). In the mid-1910s the Sanidad constantly had to make difficult choices about where to provide service. For instance, in 1916 when Ambato was first invaded by plague, public health officials were unable to carry out the rat reduction and hygiene campaign they knew was indispensable due to lack of funds. With the reduction in Guayaquil plague cases in April that year, in May the service of inspecting train passengers heading for the interior was suspended; the savings of 200 sucres per month allowed an increase in yellow fever work in the port. In February 1917, the service withdrew its anti-plague campaign in Alausí given the lack of funds to continue it. An enormous setback was suffered in October 1917 when the main offices of the Sanidad in Guayaquil were destroyed by fire—including the building itself, the records, the furniture and office equipment, and all of the serums and vaccines stored there in a "magnificent Mulford refrigerator" that had been recently imported from the United States.[39] (By a stroke of luck, the anti-plague serum was saved, because it was being stored in the cold room of the Las Peñas beer factory rather than in the Sanidad offices.) By January 1918, the service's funding was restored to a level of 15,000 sucres per month, but this was insufficient to cover the cost of an anti-plague campaign in Manabí when a new outbreak occurred there. In that case, the service managed to secure 1,200 sucres in extraordinary funds from the central government, which it considered entirely inadequate for the job at hand given that six towns were infected. To begin the campaign in Manabí it was necessary to recall the public health inspector who was carrying out anti-plague work in Babahoyo (capital of Los Ríos province), without that campaign having been concluded.[40] Clearly, simply establishing the service (and even specifying a budget, which was not always paid out) was not enough to make it operational.[41]

Following the founding of the Quito subdirectorate, complementing the national directorate in Guayaquil, there were two poles from which public health programs could emanate, each with staff, equipment, expertise, and material resources. The Guayaquil director general and Quito subdirector worked closely together across the distance. But in the mid-1910s, how did they communicate with each other to enable coordinated action? This predated the extension of the telephone service which was only connected between Guayaquil and Quito in 1920,[42] so they relied primarily on regular written correspondence, which took two days by train to reach its destination, along with brief telegraph messages when urgency demanded it. Institutional ethnography directs our attention to how the work of people is coordinated by texts, connecting their work to activities in the past and orienting them toward the future as well as connecting people across multiple spaces.[43]

The early correspondence between Sanidad Director General Becerra and Subdirector Miño is striking in how personal it is, marking an early stage in the institutionalization of this service. Their exchanges are frank and informal expressions of the problems the service faced and evoke the impression of a small, beleaguered band of public health reformers fighting an uphill battle financially, politically, and in the arena of public opinion. As Becerra wrote to Miño in November 1915, "My dear friend: Your last letter is so distressing (*desconsoladora*). How can it be that public health is the last priority? When all else is lost, at least reputation should remain: reputation of the nation, represented by the guarantees to life that all nationals and foreigners should expect. A country that does not offer these guarantees cannot prosper. . . . What to do?!"[44] The correspondence resembles an ongoing conversation between two friends. It has none of the formal tone of later letters of this kind, which reported solely on official issues—clearly mindful of leaving a written record of consultations and decision-making—and were typically addressed to the position, displacing the individual in favor of their institutional role,[45] such as "Sr. Subdirector de Sanidad," "Sr. Presidente Municipal," or "Sr. Ministro de Gobierno." Instead, Becerra's letters were addressed to "Dr. Carlos Miño, my dear friend," they mixed personal matters with official ones, and they often concluded with best wishes for Miño's wife Rosita and "su simpática heredera" ("your charming heir"), his daughter Marujita, with the diminutive "-ita" expressing familiarity and affection. When Dr. Wenceslao Pareja replaced Becerra in 1921, Miño and Pareja used the unprecedented informal pronoun "tú" in their official correspondence, showing an even greater intimacy. Indeed, they were closer contemporaries, born within a few years of each other, unlike Becerra who was fifteen years older than Miño and almost two decades older than Pareja. In addition to being coworkers in the Guayaquil Sanidad office, Miño and Pareja had also worked side by side for several weeks in an urgent disease eradication campaign during the 1913–1914 civil war on the northern coast, experiences through which they had apparently forged close bonds. These first years of the Quito office represent an era where the service was expanding its public health activities quite quickly in the country's two main cities, but the internal correspondence still showed a lack of institutionalization of interoffice relations within the service. These relations were based instead on personal bonds and trust, depending heavily on who filled the posts rather than on a more robust institutional structure.

Their correspondence also reveals the difficulties of having the central office of the Sanidad in Guayaquil while the seat of national government was Quito. The fact that Miño had previously worked under Becerra's authority in Guayaquil may have helped to keep the lines of authority clear under these conditions. Frequently Becerra asked Miño to present arguments or background information to cabinet ministers or President Leonidas Plaza (in 1912–1916, who was sometimes referred to in the correspondence as "our friend, the General") to influence their deliberations. Becerra similarly consulted with Miño to intuit the general mood of government leaders and their likelihood of supporting public health proposals; indeed, attempts to read the political landscape were a continuous part of Sanidad work.[46] Miño was increasingly well-positioned to read the institutional landscape broadly defined: he was named an honorary member of the Junta de Beneficencia in early 1919; later that year, he became president of the philanthropic Sociedad Protectora de la Infancia; in 1920, he was a member of the municipal council of Quito; and he was elected first deputy (*diputado principal*) for Pichincha province in the national legislature for the terms 1920–1921 and 1922–1923.[47]

While public health programs began to advance in Ecuador's two principal cities (see chapter 3 for Quito), how feasible was it to extend public health measures out from Quito and Guayaquil to other smaller cities or rural areas? What kind of networks of personnel and information could public health leaders harness to move their campaigns forward? Provincial capitals and cantonal seats (*cabeceras de cantón*) used locally generated resources to pay for the part-time services of municipal physicians, who combined these duties with private practices. These physicians were expected to provide some medical attention to the poor population who could not otherwise access these services and to oversee such activities as smallpox vaccination, which had long been a municipal responsibility. While the Sanidad could call on their cooperation when diseases broke out, there were serious difficulties related to lines of authority and accountability. Becerra comments on such to Miño in March 1914:

> You know from experience how completely null and void are the services provided by municipal physicians, over whom the Sanidad can never exercise the necessary authority. They are under the authority of the Municipal Councils who appoint them; and thus due to their poorly-conceived sense of self-worth (*amor propio*) . . . they feel offended in putting themselves under the orders of the Sanidad. Even the Councils feel deprived of their authority and do not offer support to this office's decisions. For this reason, and because we need employees who rigorously follow the instructions that we give—employees whom we can mobilize and even replace if necessary—I think it is necessary to create provincial subdirectors of public health.[48]

It wasn't only Sanidad leaders who found this situation frustrating. As the municipal physician in Latacunga, provincial capital of León, explains in March 1916 (when Ambato, the capital of neighboring Tungurahua province to the south, was experiencing its first plague outbreak): "I am simply a municipal physician without time for anything but local tasks, which often coincide with the arrival time of the trains" (relevant because of the need to monitor passengers and cargo to interrupt the spread of plague). He continues, "I have no personnel available to me, there is no municipal police force, the train station is distant from my office, I have no access to any kind of vehicle, and my remuneration is only 60 sucres per month."[49] Despite these constraints, he had done his best to examine any train passengers who arrived in the city, but he urged the Sanidad to establish a nationally funded public health commission to carry out any other preventive measures they might deem necessary.

Just as the Sanidad needed personnel they could depend upon, so too they needed reliable information to allow them to track disease trends and to design interventions. In this regard it is helpful to think of Sanidad physician leaders as applied scientists, which highlights their considerable dependence on data generated by others.[50] It wasn't just a question of access to this information: more often than not, they had to foster the creation of it. Then, based on their own judgement, experience, and knowledge of broader trends, they had to interpret it to predict the possible trajectory of disease. They also had to convince people of the seriousness of risk and to follow their recommendations, as they tried to influence behavior in order to prevent or limit the spread of disease.

The image of public health as a technical activity, standing apart from and looking down over society—indeed, in doing so, also generating a notion of society—can be seen in some of the initial steps that Miño took on setting up the subdirectorate in Quito in 1914. One of his first acts was to establish a statistical subsection within the office. This highlighted a central task of Sanidad work: to track trends in disease incidence. Statistical work depended in important ways on data generated by others; while the service could work to improve that data, it was not in a position to singlehandedly produce it. In his first annual report, Miño explains the importance of establishing a statistics section within the office "for the comparative study of birth and death rates in the population, in order to attend to the causes that influence the disproportion between one and another of these phenomena."[51] On examining the civil registry records—where deaths had begun to be registered following the 1900 Law of Civil Registry (another element of secularization, as it brought these records under state rather than church control)—he found it was impossible to formulate statistics about causes of death because no consistent principles guided the causes of death noted in death certificates. Taking advantage of his location in Quito, Miño met with the national director of the Civil Registry, and they came to an agreement that no death would be registered without a formal cause of death documented by either the attending physician or the subdirectorate of Sanidad if no physician had attended. He then informed both the private physicians of the capital and the directors of Quito's two hospitals of the requirement to report cause of death in accordance with the Bertillon system of nomenclature of illnesses, a copy of which he provided to them. And finally, he communicated these requirements to the president of the Sociedad Funeraria Nacional to ensure that no interment would be permitted to occur in Quito's cemeteries without the appropriate documentation.

This illustrates how Miño began to maneuver the Sanidad into a quasi-supervisory role over individual physicians and healthcare institutions in Quito, creating new requirements that they had to fulfill. It also emphasizes the challenges of having to rely on the data generated by others. To design evidence-based interventions required the Sanidad to generate new insights by bringing together dispersed data—some of it previously nonexistent—on individual causes of illness leading to death. This also meant that the Sanidad was moving toward a different vision of health conditions than that available to individual physicians, who only saw their own patients: the Sanidad began to see (and, in so doing, discursively constitute) the *population*. To advance along these lines, they needed physicians not only to use the same disease categories but also to disclose to the Sanidad their identification of any contagious diseases. While this was necessary to design timely interventions, it was also key to fulfilling Ecuador's international obligations, since the government was required by sanitary conventions to report incidence of some specific diseases to international organizations. At the same time as the Ecuadorian government had new obligations to external regulatory bodies, within the country this also realigned individual physicians' responsibility to disclose to the national Sanidad service any cases they treated of infecto-contagious diseases.

Securing that cooperation was not easy, as Becerra comments in 1915 in his annual report to the minister in regard to a typhoid fever outbreak in Guayaquil:

> It has not been possible to formulate a complete picture of the typhoid fever outbreak, because, unfortunately, and for reasons I have not been able to comprehend, the physicians of this city have not complied with the service's regulation regarding the disclosure of cases of this disease that they encounter among their private or hospital clientele. I have had to assign an employee to the task of identifying on a daily basis the cases that have occurred in the city, as confirmed by medical diagnosis: a difficult task with unsatisfactory results, but the only measure available to me to be able to order vaccination in the affected neighborhoods.

Becerra recalls that this was not the first time he had encountered this problem:

> On 24 November 1913 the Sanidad directorate sent a circular to all of the physicians of the city, explaining to them the necessity of knowing the advance of [dysentery] infection . . . in order to take the necessary measures to avoid its spread . . . but unfortunately this received the same response as the circular sent subsequently regarding typhoid fever. To what is this resistance due? I do not know, but it is regrettable to be deprived of this valuable assistance, indispensable for statistics and to better design prophylactic measures. A law making it obligatory to notify us of any infecto-contagious disease is essential. . . . The health of the collectivity is above

> any prejudices that, without any scientific basis, are rooted in an illogical conventionalism.[52]

Apparently local public health regulations, which did mandate these requirements, were not sufficient to ensure physicians' compliance, leading public health leaders to suggest that this be mandatory under national law. As I have argued elsewhere in relation to the categorization of birthing conditions in the Sanidad's records, regularizing the meaning of administrative categories as information flowed from more local to central offices was a significant challenge.[53] While only partially successful, these efforts reveal the persistent concern of this state agency with gathering and systematizing information about health conditions that would allow it to act on the population in ways informed by its unique nation-wide vision of health problems.

Consolidating Public Health as a State System and a State Idea

Sanidad leaders continued to argue for the need to have nationally funded public health employees in provincial capitals into the 1920s. The best that they could achieve, however, was that provincial delegates were appointed *ad honorem* in a few strategically located provincial capitals in 1923, still usually on a temporary basis when disease outbreaks occurred. This changed after the 1925 Revolución Juliana (July Revolution). Consistent with the consolidation of other government institutions in Quito in the post-Juliana era, the Sanidad main office was moved to Quito, and a subdirector was appointed in Guayaquil for the coastal provinces and another in Ecuador's third largest city, Cuenca, for the southern zone. The Sanidad had until then been the only national service headquartered in Guayaquil. The advance in Guayaquil's sanitation work, the elimination of yellow fever and smallpox, and perhaps, too, the incursion of bubonic plague into highland locations may have reduced the preeminence of Guayaquil in the national Sanidad structure. It is also likely that the termination of the liberal government, which had symbolized the domination of coastal interests in the presidential offices, informed the transfer of the national headquarters to Quito.

Indeed, an extensive process of organization and consolidation occurred in the Sanidad. Just a month after the 1925 Revolution, the provisional governing junta indicated its intention to have the central government share with municipalities the cost of a proper public health service in provincial capitals.[54] In August, already the larger organizational structure of the service was being changed, via the creation initially of two districts, with the idea of unifying all services under a single scientific administration. Initially, Dr. Luis G. Dávila was named director of the northern district centered in Quito, while Pareja was named director of the southern district—a large and diverse area that included both the coast and southern highlands—in this preliminary reorganization. These two directors had equal status. Half a year later, on February 23, 1926, a new Law of Public Health (Ley de Sanidad Pública) was passed to unify and coordinate public health efforts, with a further reorganization of the national territory into three zones (northern highlands, southern highlands, and coast) under a director general headquartered in Quito. The relationship with municipal governments also changed: the Sanidad service was conceived as the directive and technical organ and the municipalities as the immediate managers of the hygiene of population centers. This facilitated the Sanidad's insistence, as its director general explains to the municipal council president of Riobamba in April 1926, that "municipalities must cooperate with the Sanidad not simply in undertaking defensive projects when a threat appears, but rather in carrying out lasting, definitive programs of prevention that will ensure public tranquility and progress, on a foundation of hygiene and health. It is time for the Municipalities to understand that it is their primordial duty to dedicate their energies to the redemptive work of sanitation and hygiene of the cities, rather than projects of beautification—projects that are premature given the urgent need first to safeguard the health, welfare, and full physical development of the inhabitants."[55]

The internal organization of the Sanidad service also changed. The new director general of the service effective February 1926 was physician Pablo Arturo Suárez.[56] He was a well-respected figure, based in part on his specialist medical studies in Europe (where he was caught by the First World War, in which he served as a field medic) and his importation into Ecuador of one of the first X-ray machines for his medical practice. He also had a leading role in the Faculty of Medicine at the Universidad Central as professor of hygiene and social medicine,[57] and he was known to have administrative skills (which were recognized again in the early 1930s when he was named rector of the Universidad Central). Almost two decades after the founding of the Servicio de Sanidad, from April to July 1926 provincial delegates of Sanidad were finally appointed who reported to the regional subdirectors for each zone and through them to the director general of Sanidad in Quito. These were salaried staff positions that focused on combating contagious diseases and directing preventive health measures. These processes marked a considerable institutionalization of the service, establishing a formal structure from national director through regional subdirectors to provincial delegates, with flows of information both up and down this hierarchy.

Miño, perhaps too closely associated with the previous liberal governments to succeed to the director position, was appointed to the newly created position of inspector general of public health. He traveled widely in this capacity to inspect health conditions and establish campaigns against contagious diseases throughout the national territory. Indeed, his position fell somewhat outside the new structure of the service, as someone who traveled across the regions and had a considerable amount of independence in his role. For instance, when plague began to spread in the southern hamlets of Loja province bordering Peru in March 1926, it became urgent to study the sanitary conditions of the southern zone and establish appropriate anti-plague measures. Miño thus traveled to Cuenca to conduct an intensive training course on public health principles and practices and, based on its results, recommended personnel to staff the new regional subdirectorate of Sanidad for the southern zone. He then proceeded farther south to establish the anti-plague campaign in Loja province bordering Peru.[58]

As their internal correspondence demonstrates, Ecuadorian Sanidad leaders were very aware of the difficulties they faced in forging a personnel network within the Sanidad with clear lines of authority and accountability as well as in establishing constructive relations with other institutions. These problems were not unique to Ecuador. The first meeting of the Pan American Public Health Directors in September 1926 involved extensive and frank discussions among public health leaders from across the hemisphere about precisely these problems, where they shared their experiences and sought feedback and advice from their peers. The meeting was held in Washington, a block from the White House at the prestigious Willard Hotel (where US presidents traditionally stay on the eve of their inaugurations). The public health directors from Bolivia, Brazil, Colombia, Cuba, Chile, the Dominican Republic, Ecuador, Guatemala, Haiti, Honduras, Mexico, Panama, Paraguay, Peru, the United States, and Venezuela met for five days in late September, alternating between working sessions and social and diplomatic events such as a reception at the White House with President and Mrs. Coolidge. Chronologically, the second main topic discussed at the meeting, after a review of the Pan American Sanitary Code and modifications that might be proposed for consideration at the next Pan American Sanitary Conference, was the administrative structure of public health work in each country. Indeed, this discussion dominated three of the five working sessions of the conference.[59] While the delegates to the conference brought their own experiences and concerns into the discussion, issues that came up repeatedly included relations between institutions of social welfare and public health, relations with municipal governments (including what would be an appropriate financial contribution by municipalities toward the cost of public health campaigns), and relations with central political offices.

Suárez's oral presentation on the organization of Ecuadorian public health services emphasized the new configuration that had only been in place since the February 1926 restructuring of the service, which he felt had already produced positive results in its first six months. In particular, he emphasized the parallel organization of, on the one hand, the three regional zones of the Sanidad service, with zone subdirectors overseeing delegates in each province, and, on the other, the three regional Juntas de Asistencia Pública (previously Beneficencia) similarly overseeing subdirectors in each province.[60] These branches of state service were governed by two new laws of Sanidad and of Asistencia Pública, such that "in the entire territory no invalid remains without medical assistance." This comprehensive organization was facilitated by the recent creation of a new ministry (the Ministry of Social Welfare—directed initially by physician Isidro Ayora, who would soon thereafter be named provisional president) that oversaw both the directorates of Sanidad and of Asistencia Pública. The Asistencia Pública was charged with "problems related to assistance to the ill, to the deranged, to the unprotected elderly, and child welfare."[61]

Each provincial delegate of the Sanidad oversaw the municipal physicians that municipal governments were required to fund, who served as the "managers of local hygiene," and the law clearly indicated the obligation of each municipal government to "monitor and improve local hygiene and to indicate all possible measures, with the intervention of the Sanidad delegate of the respective province, to extinguish the illnesses that appear in the local territory."[62] The municipalities had the responsibility to collect their own statistics and pass them on to the provincial delegate, who would transmit them to the subdirector of the zone, who would in turn pass them on to the service's national headquarters, which would produce general statistics out of the data flowing to it from the most remote municipalities. Municipal governments continued to be responsible for compulsory smallpox vaccination, as they had been for many decades, including maintaining the vaccination registry. The Sanidad oversaw these activities, given the lack of staff to undertake them directly, and would attempt to correct, perfect, and modify these services to the extent possible. Similarly, the Sanidad would carry out a technical review of projects, such as the provision of potable water, sewage, and the construction of public buildings by municipalities, to correct the "inevitable errors" that smaller municipalities without sufficient technical staff might otherwise make. (These provisions considerably realigned the responsibilities of various government actors in ways that did not always proceed smoothly; see the account in chapter 4 of how this unfolded in Tungurahua province.) Half a year after the establishment of this new structure, Suárez expressed considerable optimism about the harmonious and productive functioning that it would enable.

Even within the Sanidad, however, relations could be strained. Just the previous month, Suárez had experienced a good example of this. In August 1926, Miño's report on his work organizing the southern region's Sanidad office and the Loja anti-plague campaign was unusual in being addressed simultaneously to the minister and the director general of Sanidad,[63] rather than being submitted to the director general who would then report to the minister as he deemed necessary. When Miño was appointed to his post as inspector general, he initially visualized a direct relationship with the minister, something that the new director general objected to since this would disrupt normal lines of authority. Despite this early incident, visible signs of friction were infrequent between Miño and Suárez. However, when Suárez's successor Alfonso Mosquera Narváez took over the director position (which he would hold from late 1928 until he recommended that the main office be moved back to Guayaquil in 1935—see chapter 1), working relations were more strained with Miño, possibly because Mosquera Narváez had previously worked under Miño's supervision in the Quito subdirectorate and was some fifteen years his junior. While Suárez himself was a decade younger than Miño, it is likely that his status as a respected medical researcher as well as practitioner, and the admiration he commanded as someone with European specialist medical training, situated him differently than Mosquera Narváez. The strain between Mosquera Narváez and Miño was evident in the internal correspondence of the Sanidad, even though the overall tone of that correspondence was much more neutral than in the 1910s. While this might be seen simply as reflecting interpersonal conflict, it also points to some of the tensions involved in developing a structure of personnel that could act in a coordinated way in the face of health emergencies. That is, sometimes there are built-in structural tensions between positions of authority that cannot be attributed only to individual personalities and relationships, although the latter could exacerbate them.

These difficulties were deepened by the economic instability of the 1930s, when budget reductions in the service contributed to heightened tension between Mosquera Narváez and Miño. With the support of Pan American Sanitary Bureau traveling representative John Long, Miño lobbied for the establishment of an anti-plague section within the service under his direction, while still serving as inspector general.

Mosquera Narváez objected that Miño would be unable to attend to his duties leading eradication campaigns against other diseases if he held both roles. Despite those objections, the anti-plague section was created in January 1932. Conflict came to a head when budget difficulties forced the reduction of Miño's per diem budget by 50 percent the following month, leading to several weeks in which the latter neglected to respond to official communications and orders from Mosquera Narváez (including the urgent need to initiate a new anti-plague campaign in Chimborazo to confront an outbreak).[64] In the end, Miño seems to have prevailed in these internal disputes: not only was the minister of government and social welfare persuaded to appoint him as head of the new anti-plague section while still serving as inspector general, but at Long's urging he was also appointed as temporary traveling representative of the Pan American Sanitary Bureau for the purposes of consulting regionally on plague eradication campaigns.[65] While this appointment constituted well-deserved international recognition of Miño's expertise, the resulting distractions from his core role may have impacted the Sanidad's ability to fulfill its mission in an era of significant economic stress, as Mosquera Narváez feared. Perhaps it is not surprising that these tensions surfaced more when the service was underfunded—and when the political landscape was also very unstable in the 1930s—than in the late 1920s when there was more optimism about moving forward with public health work and political and social reform.

In the 1920s and 1930s the tasks of strengthening both the state system and the state idea were ongoing projects rather than stable achievements (and indeed are likely always so). Some of the awkward internal relations generated by the growing pains of the state system could productively be seen against the backdrop of the rise of the idea of public health as a sphere in which individual rights and freedoms were sometimes superseded by a broader social interest. Just as members of the general population might be required to be isolated in a quarantine facility (whether they wanted to be or not) when they were infected with yellow fever or bubonic plague, or otherwise subordinate their personal desires or privacy to a larger public interest, so too public health physicians themselves might have to set aside their own aspirations or individual interests for the good of the collectivity. Mosquera Narváez modelled this when he voluntarily ceded the national directorship of the Sanidad back to the Guayaquil office when the port was reinfected with plague in 1935, reducing his own role from director general to subdirector in the interests of the service being able to respond more nimbly to the emergency. A different kind of example was seen when Pedro Zambrano was leading the Guaytacama anti-plague campaign: his wife was seriously ill in Quito at the time, and despite his strong desire to be at her side, he stayed in Guaytacama until he was no longer needed there. Given the nature of their work, it is not surprising that some public health leaders paid for their commitment with their lives when they fell ill with the diseases they were combatting: one of the most striking instances was the death of *all* of the medical staff confronting the pneumonic plague outbreak in Riobamba in 1939. Although he was no longer a public health official in 1945, Suárez himself suffered a massive stroke that year, which his descendants attribute to his many years of operating X-ray equipment at his tuberculosis clinic without what we would now consider appropriate protection. The stroke left him a shadow of his former self until he died a few months later.[66]

There is a difference between voluntary sacrifices and inadvertent ones, but nonetheless it may have served a legitimating function that the service itself, through the actions of some of its employees, embodied the notion of sacrifice for the larger good. That is consistent, too, with how the Sanidad saw itself as apolitical, as above and beyond politics and personal ambitions. As discussed in chapter 1, this could be seen in the service's actions during the anti-plague campaign in Guaytacama, when it showed its capacity to stand above and intervene in social conflicts. In the internal correspondence among Sanidad officials, too, it is clear that they distinguished themselves from the government: the latter was seen as composed of elected representatives who made heavily politicized statements. Hence Miño's comment to Becerra in 1915 that "the government has no problem emitting decrees that are impossible to fulfill given the lack of funds; with these decrees the government washes its hands before the public and you will no doubt be the Christ [crucified] when the public demands services that cannot possibly be provided due to the absolute lack of resources."[67]

While Miño and Becerra both seemed closely aligned politically with the second government of Plaza in 1912–1916, they did not see themselves as political actors in the same way that Plaza and other elected officials were. (This is especially striking in Miño's case, given the political positions he occupied alongside his professional role.) They saw themselves, instead, as technical experts working under multiple constraints—principal among them, inadequate funding (partly due to the decisions of elected figures) to carry out the measures that science and experience dictated.[68] In the early decades of the twentieth century, Ecuadorian physicians associated with government leadership and state institutions worked hard to position themselves and their agencies as capable of intervening beneficially in social life. As this chapter shows, they were instrumental in developing new institutional structures that facilitated administrative action in an impressive range of areas. The forging and strengthening of new images of the state, where they also played an important role, is just as significant for state formation itself and an anthropology of the state. In the context of extending public health work into domestic spaces in Quito, and out to provincial cities, the next two chapters explore what kinds of social dynamics facilitated or hindered that work.

Chapter 3

Reaching In

Waste, Water, and Public Health Services in Quito

> The work of the Sanidad is not, as it might first appear, only one of inspection and rigor, no: the mission of the Office is also intensely moral and educational. . . . Gradually, without haste or impatience, we are succeeding in inculcating in the soul of the people—with the help of the press—a certain attachment to the new sanitary practices and a certain affectionate respect for the branch's prescriptions, attachment and respect that are born naturally from the conviction of the goodness of the hygienic measures that we have managed to suggest, sometimes patiently by means of scientific popularization, sometimes with the necessary injunctions in the few cases of persistent obstinacy or reincidence against the relevant regulations. . . . Thus, the Sanidad service has deeply entered the minds of the people and has rooted itself in their habits.
>
> **—Dr. Carlos Miño, Quito-based subdirector of Sanidad, 1920**

The establishment of a stable Sanidad subdirectorate in Quito—the second location to receive permanently stationed public health staff—created the conditions for an extensive and sustained public health campaign in the capital city. The processes involved reflect the dynamics of an important urban area; in the next chapter, we turn to the rather different circumstances involved in reaching out into provincial areas of the highlands. Miño's comments above prompt the question: What were the practices that helped encourage "a certain attachment to . . . and a certain affectionate respect for" some of the public health measures promoted by the Sanidad service in Quito?

There are many excellent studies of Quito in the early twentieth century, among which the analyses by historian Ernesto Capello and historian and anthropologist Eduardo Kingman Garcés stand out for their relevance to this project, including their treatment of politics and administrative processes as well as hygiene.[1] As Kingman Garcés points out in general terms, "The various forms of ordering urban space are the expression of diverse strategies to administer populations," about which he offers a wide-ranging analysis of over a century of Quito's history.[2] Early work by Guillermo Bustos Lozano and Milton Luna Tamayo also continues to shape my understanding of life in the city,[3] and Ana María Goetschel's discussion of gendered spaces oriented my own analysis of the everyday practices of women of limited resources navigating Quito's institutional landscape.[4] Here, I add to the existing literature by focusing on how various actors engaged with the Servicio de Sanidad (Public Health Service) around problems associated with drainage, water, and waste in the city, especially highlighting how the service succeeded in positioning itself as a problem solver. It complements Kingman Garcés's analysis of the conceptual frameworks of early twentieth century hygienists and then social medicine approaches in the 1930s through a focus on the first decade of Sanidad operations in the city in the 1910s. Building on studies that examine such issues as the expansion of the sewer grid and water services,[5] this chapter provides insight into some of the everyday practices by which these external urban services became internalized—that is, brought into domestic spaces—a necessary step toward modifying intimate dimensions of behavior.

Advances in urban sanitary infrastructure were situated in ongoing and evolving relations among different levels of government. For instance, during Gabriel García Moreno's regime in 1860–1875, provincial governments' authority was strengthened (at the expense of the previous system of three districts of the national territory, which was dismantled), especially by creating new provinces and therefore expanding the number of provincial administrators as well as increasing their influence.[6] Municipal governments in turn benefited from gaining access to new mechanisms to recruit labor for public works such as road and school construction, both cornerstones of García Moreno's governing program. In the ensuing years, however, especially following the passage of the first Ley de Régimen Municipal in 1878 that extended García Moreno's initiatives, municipalities' freedom to act was constrained by restrictions on their ability to sell landholdings without national government approval and to control their own budget process, as they were only allowed to tax directly luxury items, entertainment, and animal slaughter. Capello elaborates that "the major cities of Quito, Cuenca and Guayaquil were particularly affected; their budgets were overseen not only by the provincial authorities but also by the national congress."[7] This was a period when modernization projects were sometimes funded by the national treasury, including both projects in specific urban locations (such as provision of electric lighting) and others that aimed to link up spaces (such as construction of telegraph lines and development of the postal system). An increase in monitoring of municipal initiatives and restrictions on their budgetary autonomy by the national government went hand in hand with provision of some additional resources, making these relations fraught.

This continued up to the liberal period, when a restoration of local fundraising power was welcomed after 1895. "One of the crucial pieces of the Liberal Party program concerned its support for fiscal decentralization of public works projects. The ensuing system established independent juntas empowered to organize development programs according to local needs."[8] This was not the same as returning power to municipal governments. In Quito, for instance, in May 1906 President Eloy Alfaro issued a decree that Quito's potable water, drainage, and paving should be considered national projects (*obras nacionales*) overseen by a newly created Junta de Agua Potable y Canalización de Quito, whose members would include the minister of public works.[9] As we saw, there were also ongoing tensions when municipalities were expected to take some responsibility for public health after 1908, while still having limited economic means available to them to do so. By the early 1920s, the independent juntas sometimes were seen as having gained too much autonomy. Following the 1925 Revolución Juliana (July Revolution), there was again increased monitoring by the central state, accompanied by providing additional resources that were freed up by the overhaul of national finances and budgeting processes. This occurred under the national leadership of physician Isidro Ayora, who prior to the Revolución Juliana had served on the Quito municipal council, including as its president. Ayora's government passed a new municipal code in 1929 that at the same time affirmed municipal control over daily tasks while strengthening central government oversight. Municipal autonomy was a sufficiently thorny issue in the late 1920s that the renewed Conservative Party under Jacinto Jijón y Caamaño (who would go on to become Quito's municipal president in 1934 and then mayor in the mid-1940s[10]) incorporated demands for more autonomy into its party platform.[11] Capello highlights how municipalities attempted to reestablish their control over urban planning during the 1930s, when the national government was weakened politically by rapid turnover and economically by the global economic depression.[12]

The establishment of a national Sanidad service in 1908 immediately created the conditions for interference in local autonomy, while it also created at least a potential conduit for national resources to be invested in local areas. The anomaly that a national service was headquartered in Guayaquil instead of the national capital Quito was a product of the gravity of Guayaquil's health problems but also the consolidation of its status at the end of the nineteenth century as the dominant economic center, displacing Quito. This situation points to some distinctive problems related to the identity of Quito as simultaneously the capital city and the country's "second city," an unusual circumstance in the comparative context of Latin America. This created both responsibilities and opportunities, the latter including greater central state impetus for sustaining local development.

Another important dynamic—at the interpersonal level—becomes clear in the material that follows. In the first decades of the twentieth century, Quito's city center continued to be inhabited by diverse social groups who lived in close proximity to one other. It was only in and after the 1920s that the development of new residential neighborhoods to the north of the historic city center advanced a process of spatial segregation by class. As wealthier residents built single-occupancy homes in the flatter northern environs, poorer neighborhoods began to appear to the south around and beyond the Chimbacalle train station. In the early twentieth century, the city center continued to be characterized by colonial-era buildings where an elite family might live in the upper story overlooking the street, the lower street front might have commercial establishments, and a range of other tenants might live in rented rooms facing the interior patios.[13] While the period examined here continued to be characterized by traditional relations of paternalism across classes, new urban sectors were also appearing who were not engaged in the ritualized relations of dependency that, for instance, Indigenous peasant tenants had with large landowners in the countryside. By the 1930s, the growth of middle sectors in Quito would change the urban social landscape considerably, as Kingman Garcés points out.[14] And as Bustos Lozano indicates, given the short life expectancy in Ecuador, by the late 1920s the majority of the population had been born since the 1895 Liberal Revolution,[15] a generational shift which contributed to changing social relations in Quito.

Pre-Sanidad Projects in Quito

In Quito, ongoing projects to develop urban infrastructure and municipal services, as well as the establishment of a national Sanidad office itself, occurred against this dynamic and tension-ridden backdrop. In his position as municipal hygiene director, in 1902–1903 physician Manuel Jijón Bello produced an overview of the sanitary state of Quito, pointing to overlapping and intermixed responsibilities of physicians, police, and Beneficencia institutions in such matters.[16] His study belongs squarely to the pre-Sanidad era when there was not a dedicated agency for public health. In this period, as well, physicians who worked for the municipal hygiene office shared responsibility with the public hospital for curative matters, making home visits to provide medical attention to residents without the resources to seek private physicians, while they also carried out smallpox vaccination. Their medical attention was conceived more in community terms than a focus on the individual patient in the hospital service, but it did not yet have a specific focus on contagious diseases.[17]

From the municipal services perspective, a key project to advance Quito's general sanitary environment prior to the arrival of the Sanidad service was the draining and backfilling of the Quebrada Jerusalén (Jerusalem Ravine), the last of the major creek ravines crossing the Quito valley. It ran along the Panecillo hill and served as an informal dumping ground of stagnant water, refuse, and excrement, relying on rainstorms and gravity to sweep away this waste and carry it out of the city into major rivers.[18] Once refilled, the Avenida 24 de Mayo was built over the *quebrada*. However, despite an 1899 mandate to build a drainage ditch in the Quebrada Jerusalén, funds were not freed up to do so until 1905. At that point, the looming plague scare seemed to provide additional impulse to this project, even though plague would not be identified in Ecuador until early 1908. The return of lawyer Francisco Andrade Marín to the municipal council presidency in 1904–1905 was also likely crucial for moving this project forward. A prominent figure in both municipal and national politics, while serving as minister of public works in 1884 Andrade Marín had transferred responsibility over water provision in Quito to the municipal government.[19] He had previously served in the Quito municipal council, including as its president in the late 1880s when the urban tram network was being discussed and again in 1892.[20] In that period, he also donated a lot behind the municipal offices to form a plaza (the Plaza Marín). In 1905 his interventions as municipal president were decisive, by channeling funds earmarked for other projects toward completion of the drainage canal. Capello comments that "besides making progress on Jerusalén drainage, Andrade Marín took advantage of the public health fears to conclude a series of other sanitary advances, including the organization of wastewater collection in the *centro*, paving the *centro* with cobblestones, and improving air circulation in public gathering spaces such as the military barracks and restaurant kitchens."[21]

By the time 1908 arrived, Andrade Marín had moved on to the position of municipal inspector general of health and hygiene, a post that represented one more step in a career of municipal involvement covering a quarter century. Given his established interests in urban policy, he was well aware of how relations between local and national instances of government could affect Quito's urban environment and services.[22] In 1908 in the municipal inspector role he facilitated the purchase of siphons that property owners were required to install (on his orders and those of the municipal police). The municipality had initially purchased them, and once property owners paid for them, his Office of Municipal Hygiene reimbursed the municipality for the twenty siphons, sold for 10 sucres each.[23] As he explains to the municipal police chief (*comisario municipal*): "Currently there is nothing filthier than conserving the plumbing of a house in communication with the sewage of the street aqueducts, without the modern salvation of siphons or water traps."[24]

Even before the Sanidad service was formally established in Guayaquil in November 1908, earlier that year—following the identification of plague in the port city—municipal authorities in Quito were authorized to carry out enhanced public health activities. In this context, in September 1908 Andrade Marín solicited 20,000 sucres in funding directly from the national minister of the interior to undertake sanitation projects in the capital city. He took advantage of the upcoming centenary of the first independence movement (to be celebrated on August 10, 1909) to decry the current state of the city and to point out what a bad impression it would make on foreign dignitaries when they arrived to participate in the independence festivities. Andrade Marín also hoped that there might be some way that the minister could decree this support directly, rather than having to submit it to lengthy and inconclusive discussions in Congress (reflecting one way that municipal projects might get bogged down). To support his request, Andrade Marín provides an evocative description of Quito's sanitary conditions:

> Many properties in the city drain into the open, into the streets, where, frequently, washing waste and other worse things appear. Most of the streets now have drainage installed; and what remains to be done requires neither much time nor significant expense. What has been lacking is sufficient attention to these matters. Closing [the openings onto] the principal quebradas; preventing piles of rotting garbage from accumulating in others; installing a good system of public toilets; ensuring that each drain is covered and has siphons or water traps installed; establishing the use of chimneys to ensure the renovation of air in kitchens, cellars, etc., and finally, preventing once and for all the flow of waste water from one property to another due to the city's uneven terrain. I believe only then, sir, in Quito it will no longer be so easy to die, or at least, death will come at its normal time, without being preceded, like now, by a long and uninterrupted series of well-known

> local outbreaks; after all, no one could doubt that the natural conditions of the climate are very favorable.[25]

As Andrade Marín well knew, the liberal government was planning an international exposition to celebrate independence in the Recoleta—the old Dominican horse pastures—in the Chimbacalle neighborhood, for which they had a budget of more than half a million sucres. These funds would be used to transform the Recoleta "into a fashionable park ringed by 'modern' structures," stimulating the construction of Belle Epoque chalets between the city center and the adjacent southern suburb of Chimbacalle.[26] Andrade Marín's goal was to capture some of the funds available for the centennial celebration (invested in lavish items like elegant ironwork and pavilions) for more fundamental transformations of urban space, consistent with many of his previous projects.

In addition to the municipal hygiene inspector position, at the beginning of June 1909 physician Dr. Francisco Martínez Serrano was named a subdirector of Sanidad in Quito, reporting to the director general of Sanidad in Guayaquil rather than to the municipal council (however, by 1910 he was reporting to the municipal council and Dr. Angel Sáenz in turn had been appointed to the still precarious position of Sanidad subdirector). Just a few days after taking up his post, Martínez Serrano highlights for the Sanidad director general's attention the innumerable quebradas that existed in Quito. Local residents were complaining that the recently founded national service should work to eliminate these sources of infection, but he points out that, really, they should be backfilled by the municipality under their responsibility for public works.

> As you well know, said quebradas have long served as places to deposit fecal materials and garbage. Since the city's few drainage canals also lead there, as do lavatories, the public believes that these quebradas emit miasmas and infectious winds that produce innumerable diseases in Quito, which as you know, is not true. What actually happens is that said quebradas constitute settings for the growth of germs like Eberth's bacillus and colicumunis etc., as well as the organic waste becoming hatcheries for flies that then carry those germs into houses and infect liquids such as milk and water as well as food.[27]

Martínez Serrano was working on a regulation that would require the residents to store refuse in garbage cans. He assured the director general that work was also ongoing on the water supply and drainage systems and reported that he had asked the minister to secure from the next Congress considerable funding for those projects. He also aspired to prohibit both private individuals and the municipality itself from depositing garbage in the quebradas, and instead he encouraged the latter to actively seek a location on the outskirts of the city to dispose of and incinerate garbage. He felt that with these steps the ravines would hold only soil and water which would cause no danger as sources of infection, and thus they could resolve "this danger that the residents of Quito consider to be the most important risk to their health."[28] While the residents and the Sanidad held different views on why the quebradas posed a danger, they might productively converge on a similar solution—and one in which both private behavior and public infrastructure improvements would play a role.

Indeed, in 1913 a new municipal director of hygiene increased domestic inspections to address issues of private behavior, while also advocating for significant investment by the municipal government on their side of the equation. The latter was successful in May 1913, when the municipal council agreed to commit "50,000 sucres, the quantity necessary to sanitize [*sanear*] the city, that is for construction of crematory furnaces, purchase of wheelbarrows [*carretillas*] for cleaning, repair of the city's sewers [*alcantarillados*] and installation of toilets and urinals."[29] On the private behavior side, he was distressed by the conditions that his staff were discovering when they carried out their visits. For instance, the inspection of a prominent house on García Moreno Street in April 1913, just before the Sanidad service began to intensify its labors, reveals such a case:

> This house, despite its location—adjacent to La Compañía Church—and the fact that its owner is an immensely wealthy gentleman, is undoubtedly one of the dirtiest houses in the city. In fact, there exists there a filthy chicken coop next to the bedrooms; in the corridors one can see numerous hens that foul them; the clothing of the owners and dependents are washed in the upper terraces which don't ever seem to be swept. There exists a large number of very dirty cages with their respective fowl. The kitchen is in terrible hygienic conditions, as it is not even whitewashed, and there are kept the straw mats and hides where the servants [*guasicamas*[30]] and their children sleep. Nor is the dining room a model of hygiene; there one observes an agglomeration of the most heterogeneous items and a little dog that, judging from the excrement on the chairs, must live in these rooms. The sleeping quarters of the domestic service are in perfect harmony with the preceding description: lack of ventilation, old wall hangings, spiderwebs, dirty floors, etc. On the ground floor, I will mention that in all the corridors there is an infinite number of boxes, reeds, agave fibers [*chaguarqueros*], baskets, bricks, stones, old hides, etc. That the patios release an infectious

stench, since in their siphons the excrement of all of the house's inhabitants is thrown.[31]

Various officials also continued to lobby for the backfilling of the quebradas by the municipality. In 1913, Municipal Hygiene General Inspector Jijón Bello endorsed a call by the political administrator (*jefe político*) of Quito canton for the disappearance of "these putrid concentrations which if they are not cleaned up are a threat to the neighborhood and the entire city." Jijón Bello explains further to the municipal council president:

> In this sense, my opinion, as I have previously expressed, is that the central quebradas must be prevented from becoming the focal point of all of the city's filth and to achieve this it is necessary: (1) to install toilets and garbage dumps appropriately sited and constructed; and (2) to collect solid waste and incinerate it either in appropriate furnaces or in some other way in outlying areas. In sum, Señor, I remind you of my repeated multiple reports to this effect, and I believe that complying with what has been requested, the [openings onto the] quebradas could be boarded up; until then, no.[32]

While there were ongoing efforts on these fronts, the same stubborn problems continued to preoccupy those working to advance Quito's sanitary conditions.

Sanidad Service Arrives in Quito

Dr. Carlos Miño, who arrived in Quito in August 1913 to set up a Sanidad delegation, added his voice to these ongoing efforts to address sources of infection. Born in Ambato, Miño had studied medicine at the Universidad Central in Quito, then took up a position with the Sanidad service in Guayaquil (from whence he was sent to combat the first plague outbreak in Alausí) and was later delegated to establish a more permanent Sanidad office in Quito. He also spent part of early 1914 in northern coastal Esmeraldas province addressing health crises there during mobilizations associated with that year's civil strife, an experience that deepened his knowledge of conditions across Ecuador's regions while also pointing to the lack of public health services in most of the national territory. Soon after arriving in the capital, he recognized that it would be necessary to assess the state of Quito's water supply. In this, as in so many other matters, first he needed more exact information on which to base his actions. "It is not possible, Sr. Minister [of the Interior] that we remain ignorant any longer of the quality and exact composition of this primordial element of life; judging by the multiplicity and characteristics of the infectious diseases that flagellate this city in an endemic manner, it is not too daring to suppose that, in large part, they are due to the poor quality of the water that is consumed here."[33] Thus he requested that the minister facilitate his access to the Guayaquil municipal laboratory to analyze some water samples, since in Quito it was impossible to undertake such analysis due to the lack of appropriate equipment and chemical components. And in response to the energetic political administrator of Quito canton (who in this role sometimes served as acting governor of the province in the incumbent's absence), he pointed out that the quebrada that concerned him was regularly sanitized, and if it was not a model of cleanliness this was "the fault of the superior authority, which does not supply the necessary elements for urban hygiene, obligating the nearby residents to deposit their waste in this area. To conclude, I repeat what in previous memos[34] I have told you: that for the sanitation of Quito the main factor that is lacking is money, without which every effort, every reform will not go beyond pure fantasy."[35]

It was clear to Miño that to address any of these early concerns, the cooperation of multiple levels of government and different state agencies would be required. While the behavior of residents played a role, he recognized that they could not alone effect the necessary changes. Indeed, these were demonstrations of what the ministers of the interior had argued over the previous decade: that public health was a necessary state function that went beyond what individuals could undertake, and also where their health, living conditions, and personal habits should not just be considered private matters. In the context of Quito, there was also considerable emphasis on infrastructure that would need to be provided by the municipality. Clearly the arrival of a public health delegation also raised expectations among a range of residents of the capital who mistakenly assumed that the Sanidad itself would be able to deal comprehensively with local health issues.[36] While this sometimes made it difficult to navigate the expectations for their work, it also potentially put the Sanidad in a position to negotiate between residents and various agencies. Indeed, in Miño's arguments about the need for coordination not only of individual efforts but also of different government offices, he was developing a notion of the Sanidad as that coordinator.

When Miño arrived in Quito as a delegate of the Guayaquil Sanidad headquarters in August 1913, the director general immediately authorized him to pass the Reglamentos del Servicio de Sanidad e Higiene en la Provincia de Pichincha, which Miño adapted from the public health regulations already in effect in Guayaquil (again showing the transferring of experiences and information between the two main cities). The high expectations for his work may have come in part from the summary comments he added to a printed broadsheet that communicated to the general public some of the most important new regulations. After reproducing the text of selected regulations, Miño adds:

> We have transcribed the above regulations so that the public will have an appropriate idea of the breadth of the sanitary reforms that we are going to undertake and all of the different ways that the Sanidad will be intervening in the hygienization of homes, providing this Delegation with the means deemed necessary to ensure that these regulations are faithfully followed. But as public sanitation is recognized by all as an immeasurable benefit, we expect that only in very rare cases will it be necessary to recur to the penalties mentioned herein. We must extinguish typhoid fever and other infecto-contagious diseases that unfortunately have been causing so many victims in the last few months, just as we must take steps to prevent an invasion of the terrible scourge, the bubonic plague, and since rats are the transmitters of this fearful disease, there is no scientific reason why this scourge could not infect this Capital, given the rapid means of transport [the railway]. It is necessary that we all maintain our houses and rooms in the most rigorous state of cleanliness and that we observe faithfully the prophylactic measures that the Servicio de Sanidad will opportunely indicate whenever necessary. In order to improve the sanitary state of the locality, and to protect the health and life of the inhabitants, all those of good judgment must cooperate in every possible way in order to dissipate the erroneous concepts and prejudices that exist regarding hygienic measures.[37]

Again we see the role of plague expressed here, heightening the sense of urgency to effect change. Many of the regulations required residents to alter their behaviors, but to do so in the context of increased municipal services. Indeed, the text of the regulations and the public communications that resulted from the broader project to put these regulations into effect moved back and forth between these emphases. The first article of Reglamento No. 10 stated: "All of the houses in the city of Quito that are located in streets where there are sewers or public drainage, will be supplied by their owners with the sufficient number of toilets duly connected to the public piping in the streets." The first article of Reglamento No. 12 stated: "Houses or any portions therein that do not meet the hygienic conditions to serve as lodgings, due to lack of light or ventilation or whatever other serious cause that endangers the health of their inhabitants or neighbors, will be closed temporarily or renovated by the owners." The kinds of reforms included in this Reglamento, the lack of which could motivate temporary eviction of inhabitants and closure of the properties by the Sanidad, included: "1. Provision of sufficient light and ventilation for bedrooms, rooms, shops, workshops, storerooms, warehouses, jails, barracks, pumphouses, churches and theaters. 2. Backfilling of ponds and marshes located under the floors of houses or in their patios. 3. Installation and repair of water closets connected to the public piping, if the houses face on to streets where there are sewers. 4. Repair of deteriorated floors at the entrance or elsewhere." Finally, the first article of Reglamento No. 15 stated: "The inhabitants, owners or possessors of houses situated in or around the city of Quito are required to maintain their rooms and outbuildings in clean and hygienic conditions to impede the spread of infecto-contagious diseases."[38]

To enforce these regulations, the Sanidad delegation had the right to demand entrance into any home without prior notice, a power that even the police did not have (as police officials themselves pointed out, perhaps with some envy). These inspections began to be regularly carried out in August 1913, immediately following Miño's arrival.[39] Miño chose to begin with warnings and suggestions, to "persuade [city residents] to modify their inveterate customs when it comes to the cleanliness of their houses." Tiring of the ineffectiveness of simple warnings, eight months later, in April 1914, Miño enlisted the help of the police chief so that "the force of the law makes itself felt against the property owners who, due to their habitual lethargy, threaten the health of the neighborhoods."[40] Again, the larger social impact of individual behavior was foregrounded. So too were the intersecting mandates of public health and the police, requiring cooperation between them but also revealing some jostling over who had the authority to take certain steps.[41] The 1918 creation of the public health constable (*comisario de Sanidad*) position allowed the Sanidad to assess fines independently for transgressions, but there continued to be situations requiring additional police support for enforcement of public health orders.

While this forceful prose suggests a punitive attitude toward residents, Miño distinguished between those who chose to disregard reforms that were in their power to make and those who could not comply with the regulations for no fault of their own. For instance, in January 1914 (a few weeks after the delegation was elevated to a subdirectorate), Miño commented to the president of Quito's municipal council that "it is my observation that there are very few property owners who do not wish for the benefits that the installation of toilets would bring," but that they were unable to comply with the regulations because of the elevated cost of toilets locally. He reminded the municipal officials that, having recently ordered some toilets for installation in public places, they were well aware that the low cost of these abroad bore no relation to the high cost in Quito. Miño thus requested that the municipal council order 1,000 toilets for importation and offer them for sale to the public at a moderate cost. As he concludes, connecting effective action with the legitimacy of state efforts, "If we wish the city to be sanitary and the houses hygienic, imposing obligations on the property owners, we should also offer them all facility that is within our reach so that if we must recur to sanctions under the Regulations, they will be both justified and applauded by our fellow citizens."[42] Although initially the municipal council found that ordering toilets for private buildings did not fall under its jurisdiction,[43] the next year they seem to have rethought this and ordered 1,500 toilets for sale to Quito residents at cost. While the municipality had previously worked to install public toilets and urinals, the Sanidad's extension of this program into private spaces moved this initiative to a new level. Miño framed this as enabling property owners to do what was advantageous for both themselves and the broader public.

The system of domestic inspections in principle was meant to involve monthly visits to people's homes. While the service did not in fact achieve such frequent scrutiny of urban residents' domestic space, it nonetheless had an impressive reach. For instance, the figures for 1914 show that in the three months in which figures are provided for the number of inhabitants in the houses inspected, the service inspected the living conditions of 49,263 residents of Quito, inhabiting 2,980 houses (see table 3.1). Urban censuses indicate that Quito had 51,858 inhabitants in 1906, and by 1922 its population had grown to 80,702. If we estimate that in 1914 there may have been some 65,000 inhabitants, then in just over four months of inspection all of the city's inhabitants would come under the watchful gaze of the Sanidad. While this figure is only approximate (and doesn't take into account the possibility of uneven scrutiny), nonetheless it indicates in a general way a considerable degree of monitoring of the living conditions of Quito's residents. It also likely signified an enhanced visibility around the city of the Sanidad service's activities. Infractions discovered during visits were penalized with fines and imprisonment enforced by the municipal police, based on lists of infractors provided by the Sanidad on a daily basis. The 1918 creation of the position of comisario de Sanidad (who for many years was the somewhat anomalously named Amable Viteri) permitted the Sanidad more independence in enforcing its orders. The measures imposed as a result of these inspections included, among other things, the elimination of pigsties within urban boundaries, the requirement to keep homes clean, the regulation of urban architecture, and most importantly, monitoring disposal of both household and human waste. In addition, on their visits the inspectors made note of any children who had not been vaccinated against smallpox and passed on this information to the municipality.

Table 3.1. Domestic inspections in Quito, 1914

Month	Number of houses inspected	Number of occupants
January	n/a	n/a
February	1,294	18,296
March	1,129	n/a
April	925	16,211
May	761	14,756
June	782	n/a
July	508	n/a
August	600	n/a
September	872	n/a
October	865	n/a
November	867	n/a
December	916	n/a

***Source:* Data from monthly reports of the work carried out by the subdirectorate of Sanidad for Pichincha province, LCE-1914, ASS/MNM.**

***Note*: In cell entries, *n/a* represents "not available."**

As Quito's residents were increasingly required to install toilets, sometimes existing conflicts among neighbors were intensified. Quito's colonial-era city center was built on uneven terrain that led to rain runoff from higher elevation houses to adjacent houses downhill. Neighbors had customary agreements (*servidumbres reconocidas*) to allow such drainage to cross their properties via canals. However, with the installation of toilets, some residents connected these fixtures to the existing conduits, resulting in their waste passing through neighboring properties. Although an 1888 municipal regulation had specified that "drainage pipes should not cross another's property unless metallic tubes are used,"[44] the number of interneighbor drainage conflicts that arose in the mid-1910s makes clear that passing a regulation could have little impact on actual practice without a variety of additional social processes to enable change. One petition to the Sanidad in 1914 states:

> If the use made of the drainage were only that established by the law, I would have no reason to protest. However, against all natural or legal right, by way of this canal all kinds of waste are sent through my property, an assault on the health and therefore the life itself of its inhabitants, as the employees of the Sanidad can themselves confirm, since last year this property was invaded by typhoid fever. In addition to this abuse, I have been told that these same neighbors are attempting to establish the service of toilets by this drainage system, by which they are only permitted to send rainwater.[45]

The petitioner requested that the Sanidad prevent this abuse and, through an inspection, also permit him to place a tightly woven metal screen where the two properties joined which would only permit the passage of rainwater. By necessity, the Sanidad was becoming a mediator between neighbors, as again private actions had public impacts. In this and other similar cases, the petitioner was a literate property owner soliciting support in dealing with a conflict with a neighbor.

Another illustrative conflict occurred in 1915. One resident of Quito, Leopoldo Jaramillo, enlisted the aid of the Sanidad in dealing with his neighbor Mercedes Ramírez v. de Vivanco (the lowercase "v.," for *viuda*, referred to her widowed status). Their houses were located on a central street, Carrera Esmeraldas. Miño requested an inspection of the situation by the engineer who directed the Oficina de Agua Potable y Canalización within the general directorate of public works (a section of the Ministry of the Interior). Engineer Ricardo Müller reports:

> I have examined the drains [*desagües*] of the house of Sr. Jaramillo where I have observed that the drainage of the neighboring house, situated above the level of Jaramillo's patio, crosses below the floor of one of his rooms, and as the drainage canal is made of bricks, these are saturated with the wastewater of the neighboring house, producing an unbearable stench and creating an unhealthy atmosphere capable, over time, of causing diseases. This inconvenience could be rectified in one of the following two ways: the first would be to replade the drainage canal with steel pipe or vitrified cement, extending from the patio of the neighboring house to the siphon of Jaramillo's house; and the second would be to connect the siphon of the neighboring house directly to the street plumbing, which would be the most rational in my view, since in my judgment there is no reason whatsoever that the owner of a house should have her sewage drainage in a neighbor's patio, first because this neighbor is unnecessarily inconvenienced, and second, because this system of indirect drainage is contrary to the general plan of the projected sewer system of this city.[46]

This report was sent to the subdirector of Sanidad with a copy to Ramírez, who proceeded to protest that the order to construct a new drainage canal violated her legal rights, since she had a servidumbre reconocido. Miño responded that the Civil Code gave her the right to send rainwater through this canal but not wastewater, which as Engineer Müller had found "converted the drain of this servidumbre in a true cesspool [*cloaca*] . . . in prejudice of the health of the residents of the house that receives this sewage." Miño reiterated that she had fifty days to complete the required construction.[47] Ramírez proceeded to complain directly to the minister of the interior, Modesto Peñaherrera, about what she considered to be Miño's unreasonable demands.[48] Miño then responded to the minister explaining that this was not a whim of his but rather expressed "necessities of both a private and public nature" and that the existing situation was "prejudicial not only for the property of Sr. Jaramillo, but beyond that, for the entire neighborhood since the patio has become the drain for all of the wastewater of the neighboring household."[49] What may have begun as a conflict between two neighbors grew to include several senior government officials, with Miño as the nodal point not only between the neighbors but also among them and various administrative and political officials. As the conflict escalated, the arguments about the significance of how human waste was disposed of were extended increasingly from an interneighbor inconvenience to the need to protect the health of the neighborhood as a whole.

These issues arose in part due to the distinctive terrain of Quito, whose sloping topography caused wastewaters and rain runoff to flow through neighbors' properties unless there was an adequate system of sewers (*acantarillado*). This problem was less about the provision of water itself and more about the flow of wastewaters. Because the Sanidad was a national agency, public health leaders had a comparative frame of reference and were aware of the specificity of the configuration of challenges faced in different parts of the national territory. Diverse locations required them to address distinctive issues involving specific constellations of actors and agencies in local environments. For instance, in contrast to Quito, many of Guayaquil's health problems were related to the means themselves by which water was stored and distributed. The chronic lack of sufficient potable water led the city's inhabitants to store water in open barrels, within which mosquitoes reproduced, thus contributing to yellow fever. Many other health problems were also related to the water supply, as so much of Guayaquil's housing was below street level. For instance, in 1912, typhoid fever was being spread through the potable water system because "the urban piping . . . crosses a terrain most of which is contaminated by organic infiltrations of all kinds." There was an urgent need to "select the most adequate means to conserve its purity [of water], now that work will begin on the new provision of potable water, choosing a spring that satisfies in both quantity and quality, the needs of Guayaquil, collecting and distributing this primordial element of life, without which hygiene is impossible, in tanks and pipes scientifically constructed and rationally located, so that never again will it occur that the cisterns of the potable water system are at the foot of a hospital."[50]

The British company White was contracted to undertake a thorough renewal of the sanitation infrastructure in Guayaquil, laying new water pipes, sewers, and drainage and paving the streets. When the White company began its work on the potable water infrastructure in Guayaquil, its excavations themselves triggered a disease outbreak. "The typhoid fever epidemic has appeared preferentially in certain neighborhoods of the city, areas that lack any kind of drainage. The excavation of soil in these streets, necessary in order to lay the new water main, has brought to the surface all of the bacillary flora deposited in the layers of soil, where the residents dispose of their feces and all manner of waste, since in those streets there is no sewer network of any kind and the so-called hygiene service is the most primitive and deficient one could possibly imagine."[51] Still, the installation work was unavoidable, given the existing state of the pipes, which led to a chronic state of contamination—a situation that was made worse by the inadequate water supply, which only flowed for a few hours a day. "In many areas of the city, without drainage, for lack of any alternative the residents dump in public thoroughfares the waste of the healthy and ill alike. The pathogens that are suspended in these liquids filtrate easily into the soil, where they encounter the water pipes that, since they are ruptured in many sections, allow all the elements that permeate the surrounding soil to easily pass through, under the influence of the difference in pressure that exists due to the fact that the pipes are empty for 18 hours a day through the entire urban network."[52]

In high-altitude Quito, built on uneven terrain, the problems had a different cause: the slopes of the city caused drainage conflicts as wastewaters generated in one household crossed the properties of neighbors. While residents could attempt to install barriers that only permitted water to pass (rather than solid waste), connection to a proper municipal system of sewers was a more effective solution, given the germs that this water could carry. As with other issues, there was a need for improved municipal services, but there was also a need for someone to mediate in these disputes between neighbors, and sometimes to advocate for them before municipal actors.

In becoming a mediator, the Sanidad also had to present itself as a neutral and fair agency, above local stakeholders. Thus the service was at pains to say that its agents inspected the homes of both the wealthy and the poor, with the difference that they tended to be more lenient with those who could not afford expensive renovations. As Miño argues in his annual report for 1917–1918, "I have placed great care in ensuring that the law and regulations are applied wherever they are necessary, without regard to fear or favor, but that has not meant proceeding with equal exigency for the wealthy and for those people who barely sustain themselves with a small property or a workshop with miniscule revenue; for the latter I have made concessions, when it comes to costly repairs, but not when it is simply a question of cleanliness and good customs."[53] Miño's insistence that his office was especially demanding of the wealthy indicates his concern to demonstrate that not only was the broader social interest above the individual rights and freedoms of the poor, but the wealthy, too, had to subordinate themselves to this. Even more so, in fact, since they were more likely to be the owners of properties that housed tenants as well as their own families or businesses with numerous employees and dependents. A case in November 1914 illustrates this, when Miño ordered that a resident be judged and punished for the infraction of not connecting his house's drainage pipes to the public sewer system, despite having been ordered to do so within a reasonable period of time.[54] The penalized individual was prominent Quiteño Abelardo Montalvo, a former president of the Chamber of Deputies (Congress).

The system of domestic inspections was quite effective in some regards. Perhaps most impressively, in the period from August 1913 when Miño arrived in Quito through the end of 1918, the Sanidad subdirectorate managed to insist on—or, more accurately, facilitate—the installation of more than 3,500 toilets and urinals in private homes and public buildings in Quito.[55] In accordance with the Reglamentos de Sanidad, the owners of homes with access to the public sewer system were required to install modern toilets, with the aim of reducing, in particular, the threat of typhoid fever, one of the most common infectious diseases that contributed to urban mortality and morbidity in Quito (indeed, it was this disease that Miño initially went to Quito to address in mid-1913). Typhoid fever was spread by flies that landed on the waste of sick individuals and then touched food or water consumed by others. However, the ability of the Sanidad to insist on the installation of toilets depended on more than just domestic inspections, or even property owners' willingness to make upgrades. This depended, too, on whether the municipal government had installed sewer and drainage systems and whether running water was available. It also depended on the availability of hygienic fixtures for purchase in the city at a reasonable price.

When they were cited for violations of public health regulations and were required to install these improvements within a given period, many property owners objected that they could not afford the required installations, which were to be made at their own expense. One solution was to provide them with a longer time period before fines would come into effect. But more importantly, the public health service encouraged the municipality to import large numbers of toilets, which were provided to residents at cost. As mentioned, at Miño's recommendation the municipality imported toilets to provide them to local residents. In November 1915, when the toilets ordered from an export firm in New York arrived, all 1,500 had already been reserved and paid for by Quito property owners. The largest order, totaling 12 fixtures, was reserved by César Mantilla, owner of Quito's Nuevo Hipódromo horse racetrack as well as the newspaper *El Comercio*.[56] Previously, in 1912 the municipality had imported 80 toilets for installation in public buildings and in public areas of the city (such as in the 24 de Mayo neighborhood).[57] Later, the 1922 Congress permitted Quito's Junta de Embellecimiento (Beautification Board, another independent junta) to invest part of their funds in the importation of hygienic fixtures to be sold to the public at cost, although these did not actually arrive in Quito until 1925. In the same period, the municipality ordered from abroad another shipment of toilets costing 100,000 sucres in the hopes that by this means toilets would be made available at a reasonable price to all city residents.

In December 1917, in support of the efforts of the Sanidad subdirectorate, Quito's municipal police chief issued a blanket order that all property owners who had not yet installed toilets were required to do so.[58] In the following months this decree ran up against yet another obstacle: there were no more water meters available to city residents, and without water service, toilets could not be installed. Following a suggestion from the Sanidad subdirector, the municipality agreed in November 1918 to allow the installation of running water without meters in the interim (just until more of these items arrived), at the moderate set price of 1 sucre per month for water for domestic uses, with higher rates assessed on larger consumers, such as industrial establishments, bakeries, and the like.[59] In addition, any new constructions to be carried out in the city had to include installation of hygienic services and comply with public health requirements concerning the construction materials used, amount of ventilation and natural light, and so on. Effective November 1917, Reglamento No. 8 required that construction plans be approved by the subdirectorate of Sanidad as well as the municipality to ensure compliance with these requirements.

Although the subdirectorate could insist upon the installation of toilets and running water in those houses with access to municipal services, it turned out that this did not guarantee that these amenities were made available to all residents of a building. In 1918, some situations of this kind were reported:

> We have determined . . . the number of urinals and toilets that must be installed in proportion to the residents, requiring that they be installed in accessible locations and that they remain open and functioning properly at all hours of the day and night for the service of the inhabitants who have the right to use them. As there are people who, having installed this equipment only to avoid fines, keep them locked—because they cannot conceive that such decent apparatuses could be dedicated to such lowly ends—it has been necessary to proceed energetically to obligate them to use the toilet even by means of repeated fines. A similar situation has arisen, with similar procedures followed, when it comes to running water (whose installation is simultaneous), as some owners, due to miserliness or whim, will not concede their use to their tenants.[60]

Indeed, the archival documents show that property owners were regularly fined if they did not allow their tenants to use toilets and running water, or if they raised rents substantially in exchange for use of these services. Most often the Sanidad subdirectorate found out about these cases because tenants asked the service to intervene on their behalf. In addition to functioning as a mediator between neighboring property owners, the Sanidad increasingly began to also fulfill this role between urban residents of different classes living in close proximity.

In addition to warnings, fines, and sometimes even imprisonment, the Sanidad also used the procedure of closing buildings temporarily (*clausura temporal*) until their sanitary conditions were improved. This procedure began to be carried out regularly in 1918, and the numbers from 1919 show that there was an average of two private homes closed per month for these reasons. In addition, in 1918 the parsonage (*casa parroquial*) of San Blas was closed temporarily,[61] and the municipal jail suffered the same fate. Perhaps the most celebrated closure for public health reasons affected the railway station in Chimbacalle, which had disastrous sanitary conditions that no government agency had previously been able to compel the foreign company to rectify. It was demolished and completely rebuilt before being inaugurated anew in May 1920.

What can be observed here is a systematic effort to eliminate any excuses that residents and especially property owners might have had for not following public health regulations. But there is more: the Sanidad positioned itself as a mediator between landlords and tenants and between property owners and the municipal government as it took on a problem-solving role in negotiating access to hygienic fixtures. The municipality had not only the ability to raise revenue but also the right to tax-free import of goods for its needs, which both lowered costs and speeded the arrival of goods that might otherwise be subject to months of delay in the customs warehouses in the Guayaquil port.[62] This all occurred despite the considerable diversion of merchant vessels to serve the war effort in Europe in the 1910s, interfering with international trade.

The result of these processes was the transformation of both the face of the city and the intimate practices of its inhabitants. The plans for all new constructions required approval from the Sanidad before work could go ahead, and often the owners were required to install a different kind of flooring or additional drains or toilets. And the florid descriptions of urban homes full of the excrement of livestock and of streets with sewage running down them began to be replaced by accounts of a drainage system with each house connected to the grid and with hygienic services throughout (although, again, this extended only so far as the municipality's program of water provision and sewers). The installation of toilets in particular resulted from state agents entering into the private sphere and regulating the outward manifestation of some of the most intimate bodily functions. While there was clearly some resistance to these measures, it was mostly expressed in terms of the cost or unavailability of these fixtures, and the Sanidad moved systematically to eliminate these objections. It should be noted that this effectiveness was limited to Quito, as many of the provincial capitals did not have the necessary sewage disposal systems and running water to permit similar modernization until later decades.

If there is any doubt that this involved a campaign of cultural reform as well as infrastructure expansion, Miño sets the record straight. Expanding the quotation that opened this chapter, Miño argues in 1920:

> The work of the Sanidad is not, as it might first appear, only one of inspection and rigor, no: the mission of the Office is also intensely moral and educational, especially in its relations with the popular classes, uneducated and therefore little disposed to concern themselves with the duties of hygiene and sanitation. Gradually, without haste or impatience, we are succeeding in inculcating in the soul of the people—with the help of the press—a certain attachment to the new sanitary practices and a certain affectionate respect for the branch's prescriptions, attachment and respect that are born naturally from the conviction of the goodness of the hygienic measures that we have managed to suggest, sometimes patiently by means of scientific popularization, sometimes with the necessary injunctions in the few cases of persistent obstinacy or reincidence against the relevant regulations.

> The courteous visit, the delicate notice, the opportune warning, the polite reminder and finally the penalty by the Comisaría de Sanidad work together to gradually establish a preventive-punitive system: such that we begin by warning as is customary, and only in extreme cases in which it is necessary to act decisively and energetically, have we arrived at the other extreme: punishment, which consists generally in a fine and rarely in prison. Thus, the Sanidad service has deeply entered the minds of the people and has rooted itself in their habits.[63]

The largest number of archival documents regarding the installation of toilets and associated processes in Quito were found for the decade of the 1910s. This period saw a considerable extension of municipal services, with a particular push in their development in 1916. In October 1915 Congress had returned to the municipal council of Quito its responsibility for the "service and construction of potable water, drainage, and paving" for the Quito canton, restoring municipal control over these activities with their associated budgets.[64] To this renewed responsibility and resources may have been added the impetus of the urgency generated by the 1916 infection of Ambato by bubonic plague, which seemed to suggest that Quito would be next if the sanitary conditions were not quickly improved. Such ambitious projects often required a sense of crisis to propel them forward.

Completion of Quito's tram system in 1914 and improved drainage across the city also helped prompt new investment in the plains to the north of the colonial city center, with the beginning of land purchases by investors grouped in the Anglo-French syndicate.[65] When they proposed the coordinated development of a new neighborhood in this area in 1919, a sewer system was incorporated into the planning from the beginning, which gave the extension of these services into new (and flatter) areas a different character than their construction in the old neighborhoods. The municipal drainage system in Quito's core was largely completed by 1922,[66] although intermittent archival documentation continued to be generated around these processes until about 1927.

Infrastructure investments by the municipality were crucial to the expansion of the grid. The ability of the Sanidad to serve as a helpful mediator to ensure the rights of tenants against landlords and neighbors against neighbors as well as to facilitate property owners' access to municipal services and fixtures was also key to how these services were internalized within private property and domestic spaces. Generally speaking, the provincial level of jurisdiction was less evident in how these processes unfolded in Quito. It became more important outside of Ecuador's main cities after the 1926 creation of provincial delegations of

Sanidad throughout the highlands and coast. The next chapter explores the different dynamic of the sometimes awkward expansion of public health personnel and programs in one highland province.

Chapter 4
Reaching Out

Extending Public Health in Tungurahua Province

When director general Pablo Arturo Suárez presented the new structure of the Ecuadorian Sanidad service to other national public health directors in Washington in September 1926 (see chapter 2), on the one hand he highlighted the respective responsibilities of provincial Sanidad delegates and municipal councils (and the physicians the latter employed). On the other, he described the parallel structure at the provincial and national levels of the Sanidad and Asistencia Pública agencies, both overseen by the new Ministry of Social Welfare. While he expressed optimism for the harmonious functioning of this system, examining a specific local case can reveal the points of pressure that could make it difficult to advance public health activities, underlining the frailty of the processes explored in this book.

The province of Tungurahua is situated in the central highlands between Chimborazo to the south and León (later, Cotopaxi) to the north. To the west it borders Bolívar province, and to the east lies the Amazon region, or Oriente. The territorial extension was relatively small—only 1.29 percent of the national territory[1]—and the fact that 6.7 percent of the national population lived in the province in 1942 gave it by far the greatest population density of any province in the country (double the average population density in the highlands, which itself was almost double the average population density in the coastal region). The National Office of Statistics estimated in 1942 that about 19 percent of the province's population lived in urban areas (over half of them in the provincial capital Ambato), while 81 percent lived in rural areas. Despite those relative proportions, with its population of just over twenty-one thousand in 1942, the provincial capital Ambato was the sixth largest city in the country.[2]

In the early twentieth century, Ambato became an increasingly busy commercial center, especially following the inauguration of the Guayaquil-Quito Railway. In the decade from 1909 to 1919, the amount of commercial capital in circulation (*capital en giro*) more than doubled, placing Ambato at the top of all central highland cities (in the provinces of León/Cotopaxi, Tungurahua, Chimborazo, and Bolívar) with 38 percent of all such capital in the region.[3] By 1922 there were two textile factories in Ambato, which together employed between four hundred and five hundred workers, many of whom lived in the rural environs of the city, and about 30 percent of whom were women. The city had many family owned leather workshops and shoemakers, which saw a gradual differentiation in the early twentieth century as some tasks were mechanized in a central location and others were sent out on a piecework basis (*trabajo a domicilio*). There were also numerous small food businesses. Tungurahua's agricultural production supported several large grain and flour mills in Ambato, and the region's fruit orchards supplied both markets in Ambato and trade to other provinces. The three market plazas in Ambato that existed in 1890 had grown to five by 1920, and in the year 1931, 605 permits were issued to market vendors (primarily women). While the province had been known for its population of *arrieros*—mule drivers engaged in trade between Babahoyo (to the west in the coastal region) and the highlands—these declined in number after trade routes were reorganized once the railway was completed in the first decade of the twentieth century. Another group of traders grew, however: *shigreros* were traders who came from rural areas as well as from Ambato (but without kin ties with the landowner-merchants who had been dominant in city trade in previous decades), who expanded their trade in the highlands of items from the coast (products imported by Guayaquil firms, national manufactured items, and coastal foodstuffs such as sugar and rice) while also moving highland leather and agricultural products to the coast. Together with a new group of foreign merchants (Italians, Arabs, and Chinese), these two commercial groups increasingly displaced the old landowner-commercial businesses that had previously dominated commercial life in Ambato. This city was in a period of commercial and industrial expansion in the 1910s, 1920s, and beyond, with intensifying trade with other regions stimulated by railway construction.

Sanidad Leaders Visit Ambato

In late 1913, the delegate of Sanidad for Pichincha province and, by extension, the north-central highlands, Dr. Carlos Miño, visited Ambato with his assistant from the Quito office, Dr. Nicolás Baca. As Miño was at the time a delegate in Quito of the Guayaquil Sanidad office, Baca was named his subdelegate in Ambato for the purposes of heading up a temporary Sanidad office there, staying behind for a time to maintain the activities established by Miño. That year plague had infected a highland location for the first time during the outbreak in Alausí, Chimborazo province, immediately south of Tungurahua. Miño's first act following his arrival was to connect with the Tungurahua provincial governor, who convened a meeting with the Ambato municipal council president, the chief of police, and Miño. They all agreed to cooperate within the scope of their attributions in the hygiene campaign to be undertaken, including by ensuring that it could proceed "without the resistance and opposition that always arises whenever old and engrained customs and practices must be uprooted."[4]

The activities undertaken on this visit are illustrative of the structure of public health work at the time. Miño asked the police chief to order that all residents, within forty-eight hours, clean their lodgings, dispose of garbage, and remove any disease-ridden animals (*animales nocivos*) from their properties. Flyers were distributed to promote smallpox vaccination as well as anti-plague vaccination (the latter for anyone traveling to infected regions). Miño printed and distributed relevant public health regulations, which had been adapted from the Quito and Guayaquil rules to meet the local circumstances. Miño and Baca also inspected the hygienic conditions of public establishments of all kinds (restaurants, bakeries, slaughterhouses, etc.) to ensure that they met the necessary standards of cleanliness for the hygienic production of food items. Orders were emitted detailing various repairs and renovations that were required within a specified timeline at these facilities. With the assistance of public health staff from Guayaquil, a small disinfection brigade was formed to "attack" areas infected with typhoid fever. A rat-hunting crew was also assembled, who used traps and poison sent from Guayaquil "to fight unceasingly against these rodents, that cause so much harm to man and that have multiplied in an extraordinary way both in the city and its environs."[5] This proliferation was a bad omen for the service's aspiration to prevent a plague outbreak.

Among the many deficiencies Miño and Baca identified in Ambato was the "terrible state of street and plaza cleaning, which is undertaken at inadequate times and in such an incomplete way that waste and garbage is left piled up in the corners, creating mounds of organic materials, fearsome foci of morbid germs that threaten public health and speak very poorly of the culture and advancement of the city." Miño immediately contacted the municipal council president, asking him to order a change to the garbage collection regime, including a new predawn collection time of four to six in the morning, "as per the usual practice in all other cities." While the municipality had set aside 6,000 sucres for public health projects, they needed authorization from the minister to expend these monies in acquiring six carts and the necessary draught animals to pull them. That is, although they had permission to establish new taxes to create funds for initiatives of this kind, they still needed approval to spend those funds. A temporary office for the subdelegation was set up in a space loaned for this purpose within the provincial Gobernación building.

As this visit indicates, there were multiple institutional actors whose efforts needed to be brought together to begin to address public health issues, coordinated under the direction of the Sanidad service—despite there not yet being a permanent delegate in the city or province. At this time, there were a number of important administrative positions that were directly appointed by the national government: national cabinet ministers, provincial governor, canton-level political administrators, and parish-level political lieutenants. The municipal government, in contrast, was elected and brought together a disparate group of local actors who might pull in different directions than appointees of the national government. Miño had to get both municipal and provincial actors working together to make some headway on public health. In establishing new services in Ambato—which was correctly identified as a strategic site of intervention for the anti-plague campaign—experience from elsewhere was drawn upon in adapting public health regulations from Guayaquil and Quito, supplies were brought from Guayaquil, and public health staff traveled from both cities to assist. Five years after the agency's founding, Sanidad personnel and experience were beginning to circulate around the national territory, although many locations still remained outside their circuit.

Ambato received more concentrated attention during the bubonic plague outbreaks in and after 1916. Still, these were considered extraordinary and urgent measures, involving temporary Sanidad campaigns rather than representing a regular component of the Sanidad's functioning. In his capacity as subdirector of Sanidad for Pichincha province and the north-central highlands, Miño might send extraordinary commissions to address specific problems—for instance, in 1921 an outbreak of varioloid in Baños to the east of Ambato led to a public health expert (but not a physician), Manuel Gándara, traveling there to lead a campaign of obligatory vaccination. This required permission from the minister to extend the existing urban health regulations into more rural areas as well as a ministerial order to the political administrators in the cantons to facilitate Gándara's work. In other words, there was no existing process or structure in place that would enable this kind of activity.[6]

The year 1926 was a watershed moment for the scope of Sanidad work in the provinces. In the second quarter of the year, permanent delegates of Sanidad were appointed in provincial capitals. Dr. Luis Joaquín Martínez was appointed to this post in Tungurahua. The incorporation of additional regional spaces into Sanidad work led to both a greater presence of higher-level officials in discussions with local authorities about public health issues and an intensification of everyday sites where the new provincial delegate's responsibilities intersected with other institutions and medical practitioners in Ambato, generating additional points of potential friction in local health-related initiatives.

As the new structure was being implemented, national authorities also visited provincial capitals. In late January 1927, director general of Sanidad Dr. Pablo Arturo Suárez made an inspection visit to Ambato. His comments to the municipal council president demonstrate the increase in technical knowledge about public health as well as the evolving structure of accountability. Following his congratulatory comments on the municipality's recent efforts to install public toilets, Suárez provided extensive guidance on the water system under construction, upon which any toilet service necessarily depended. Based on the current population of Ambato (about fourteen thousand residents at the time), Suárez calculated that the city would need 840,000 liters of water each day, which would require an approximate surface area of 374 square meters of filtration; however, a mere 150 square meters were in construction, which would only produce 350,000 liters of water per day. His comments included considerable detail about how the filtration system worked and why additional tanks were needed. He also recommended building the water system in such a way that chlorination could be added once finances permitted. He reminds the municipal council president:

> Every project of this kind should always be subject to a technical review, not only from an architectural and engineering point of view, but also from a hygiene perspective. Otherwise, these projects will never offer the anticipated result and the residents' hopes will be disappointed and municipal funds wasted, undermining all the sacrifices made. For these reasons, the Law orders that no project of this class can be carried out without technical studies of the plans and material constructions receiving the approval of the directorate of Sanidad. The responsibilities of the leaders are hereby clarified via these opportune observations I provide to you.[7]

As this indicates, the relationship between the municipality and the national Sanidad service was changing with the appointment of permanent Sanidad delegates in each provincial capital and with the new Ley de Sanidad that redistributed responsibilities between various relevant parties. This point was brought home by Suárez's observation that Ambato's municipal physician was almost completely derelict in his duties as they were redefined under the new law. As Suárez explains, "The Municipal Physicians were created, according to the current Ley de Sanidad, to fulfil the role of Directors of Municipal Hygiene in close relation to the Delegates of Sanidad. Thus, they are responsible for the control, direction, reforms, in consultation with the Delegate, of everything related to food hygiene (markets, groceries, milk provisioning, beverages, food production facilities, pharmacies, etc.), with everything related to urban hygiene (housing, public and private buildings, water service, public and private drainage, garbage collection and disposal, etc.), with everything related to municipal health statistics and smallpox vaccination." And nonetheless, to his surprise, he reports:

> I have yet to see a single document, report, statistic, or numerative list that outlines [the municipal physician's] work; I have not seen a single response to the office of the Delegate; I am not aware of any consistent work of monitoring, of reforms, of constant coordination between the Municipality and the Sanidad. It is necessary in the interests of the population itself, that Municipal Physicians commit themselves to a dedicated, enthusiastic, and correct labor. For now, I ask the illustrious Council to insinuate to the Municipal Physician that he take his duties more seriously and to obligate him to work, from this day forward, in agreement with the Regulation and the schedule determined by the Office of the Delegation, under its immediate control and direction, as occurs here [in Quito] and in other cities.

Finally, to better facilitate communication and coordination with the delegation, Suárez requested that the municipality provide space for the Sanidad office in either the municipal building or another conveniently located one. In the end, office space was provided in the provincial Gobernación instead, where it may have been easier to arrange given that the Sanidad service and provincial governor were both linked in a direct line to the national government.

The final section of Suárez's comments updated the municipality about advances in the research the Sanidad was carrying out about plague transmission, which was rapidly increasing their knowledge about how the disease spread in Ecuador. Ambato's residents certainly were familiar with both plague and plague elimination campaigns, given significant outbreaks in the city in 1916 and 1923. Suárez explained to the municipal council that it was specifically where the *cheopis* flea was prevalent that plague outbreaks occurred, and that this flea was present both in and around Alausí and in Ambato, two areas that had proven to be stubbornly susceptible to plague outbreaks.

> This is, clearly, a city infested with plague, and in periods when the *cheopis* flea arrives at an index superior to two per rat, human plague explodes without any need for cases to arrive from elsewhere: such is the current scientific principle supported by all the Epidemiology of this disease. As a result, this town is always in danger of being invaded by plague, any time the proportion of fleas increases. Based on these principles, I put in place a campaign to try to impede the return of the plague. . . . I believe that if the measures specified by the Delegate of Sanidad are followed with great care, it would be possible to contain the excessive multiplication of this insect.

Suárez urged the municipal leaders and the municipal physician to step up their efforts in the general work of sanitation, including collection and disposal of garbage and all the other measures that had been indicated, especially during the upcoming months of greatest danger (from February through April). If these measures were overlooked due to the municipality's confidence in having tamped down the plague since the previous July, Suárez predicted that "you will find yourselves again facing mounting costs and observing the enormous anguish and desolation caused by the invasion of that terrible scourge."

As Suárez's comments illustrate, one of the distinctive features of Sanidad work, informed by experience both over the previous two decades and in a variety of geographic spaces, was its officials' ability to contextualize projects and activities in a longer planning horizon. They could predict when plague was likely to flare up again and knew it would be more costly to address if preventive work was not carried out in advance. They also understood that an ambitious infrastructure project like a water system should be built in such a way that it not only provided sufficient water for current needs but also could be expanded in scale in the future as well as for chlorination to be added when feasible.

This broader perspective was clear in a discussion in which Suárez engaged over the following weeks about the water system. Ambato's engineer in charge of the work, Lunemburg, objected to Suárez's appraisal of how much water the city's residents would need, an assessment that underlay his design of the smaller-scale system that Suárez had criticized. Lunemburg claimed that even the twenty liters per capita per day of water he had planned for might be too much, since "there are few baths and toilets in use, and in the outlying neighborhoods the residents don't use much piped water." Suárez counters bluntly:

> This makes no sense to me. If water is provided to a population it is not with the intention that the inhabitants continue with the same rutinary habits of not using much water, but to the contrary, we hope to implant, intensify

> and multiply hygienic services, such as baths, toilets, irrigation, etc., and that with each day, habits of hygiene and cleanliness are more deeply rooted and extended, which will demand an ever greater supply of water. To suppose that Ambato will never grow beyond its 14,000 residents, that these will never need more baths, toilets and hygienic services than what they currently have, and that those who live in the city's outskirts will not use more water in the future than they do now with their limited, antiquated and antihygienic customs, is to not view the potable water project from the perspective of hygiene and health, but only from the narrow point of view of the rushed completion of a project that, being as it is of outmost importance, should not be celebrated until it has arrived at its happy conclusion, defined under much broader criteria than those used by Señor Lunemburg.[8]

Suárez had previously offered the assistance of engineer G. Noroña, the national director general of public works, and Ambato's municipal council president took up this suggestion in early March. By the end of March, Noroña had inspected the work and agreed with Suárez's initial assessment. Likely Noroña's inspection visit is what spurred Lunemburg to contradict so energetically the Sanidad's critical assessment. In addition to technical comments about the extension of the project, Noroña also points out the importance of relying on specialist advice and institutions collaborating effectively: "The current organization of special services, like those of hygiene, etc., has been legally instituted with authorities in each area; it is therefore imperative that there be reciprocal and harmonious collaboration among the institutions that have the same objective: to work in support of the improvements that guarantee the well-being of all, and to carry out the projects conducive to this end."[9]

The assertion of Sanidad authority over other institutions in provincial contexts clearly did not occur smoothly. This was even more true when it was in the hands of the provincial delegate rather than more senior officials from Quito. One can easily read in the documentary evidence the increasing frustration of the delegate, which both was the product of and likely itself contributed to the strained relations between the Sanidad and other agencies and officials. The Sanidad director general had a certain distance from local relations (even when he was from the region, as Suárez was) and could marshal the authority of his office as the leader of a national agency. Suárez also had specialist medical training in Europe, strong ties to the university, and an extensive research record. The provincial delegate, however, was much more immersed in local social relations in Ambato as a practicing physician in the city.

Provincial Sanidad Delegate Takes Up His Role

Luis Joaquín Martínez was born in Ambato in 1891. The extended Martínez family was well-known in the region. Luis's grandfather, lawyer Nicolás Martínez Vásconez, had served in many public positions in the second half of the nineteenth century: political administrator of Ambato, both congressman for and governor of León province (which included Tungurahua until this region was elevated to provincial status in 1860), and vice president of Congress in 1857. Conservative president Gabriel García Moreno went on to name him governor of Tungurahua, and he was elected congressman for Tungurahua in 1869 and 1871. He served as a member of the Supreme Court in 1876 and was again elected congressman for León in 1883. Nicolás Martínez Vásconez and his wife Adelaida Holguín had numerous children, the eldest of whom was Ricardo Martínez Holguín, a physician, who fathered future Sanidad delegate Luis Joaquín Martínez. Ricardo had several well-known brothers (the uncles of Luis Joaquín), including painter and writer Luis Alfredo Martínez Holguín (1869–1909), who served as secretary of education under president Leonidas Plaza and founded the Colegio Normal de Agricultura in Ambato (he married Rosario Mera Iturralde, the daughter of writer and politician Juan León Mera, who among other things wrote the lyrics to the national anthem). Another brother, Augusto (1860–1946), was a scientist of broad interests who conducted geological studies, worked in the Observatorio Astronómico in Quito, and taught chemistry. He fought in the Liberal Revolution and later served as acting governor of Tungurahua. A younger brother, Nicolás, became known as the father of *andinismo ecuatoriano* (mountaineering). These were the prominent uncles and extended family of the first delegate of Sanidad in Tungurahua appointed after the new Ley de Sanidad expanded the public health system in 1926.

Luis Joaquín Martínez had begun medical studies in the Universidad Central in 1908, part of an expanded cohort of first-year students: thirty students enrolled (three times the average cohort in previous years), but he was one of only ten who graduated in 1915 without interruption to their studies.[10] He set up a practice in Ambato soon after graduating and thus had been practicing medicine for about a decade when he was appointed to his position as provincial delegate. The best data we have about the numbers of practicing physicians in the area is from 1909 and 1941,[11] leaving 1926 when Martínez was appointed as an interim point for which we can estimate. In 1909, around the time he began his medical studies, there had been four physicians in Ambato. By 1941, there were twenty physicians in all of Tungurahua province. In 1926, there were likely no more than ten physicians in Ambato.

During Martínez's term as Sanidad delegate, numerous areas of tension surfaced around public health activities. One area of chronic strain was between the Sanidad and the Asistencia Pública. As Suárez explained in 1926 at the conference of public health leaders in Washington, the new laws of Sanidad and Asistencia Pública created two parallel agencies to deal respectively with preventive measures and disease eradication campaigns, on the one hand, and curative and social welfare programs, on the other. One site where representatives of these two institutions interacted was in provincial hospitals, which were managed by the provincial subdirector of Asistencia Pública with the exception of the contagious diseases ward, which was under the supervision of the Sanidad delegate. In the Ambato hospital, the first documented signs of friction appeared in early 1928, when the *sala de aislamiento* (isolation ward for contagious diseases) was being installed. The tensions between the local Asistencia Pública and Sanidad leaders were such that the Sanidad delegate went to great lengths to avoid having to communicate directly with the provincial subdirector of Asistencia Pública. This led to a convoluted process where the delegate wrote to the Sanidad director general in Quito, who either communicated to the subdirector of Asistencia Pública back in Ambato or communicated to the national director of the Asistencia Pública agency, who passed information, requests, or orders on to the subdirector. As the Sanidad director general points out, it would have been much more streamlined for Martínez to speak directly to the subdirector: "The obvious solution would be that you communicate directly with him, surrendering any selfishness or pride in the interests of duty and the public good."[12] Apparently, even before the installation of the isolation ward, there was already a strained relationship between the provincial Sanidad leader and his Asistencia counterpart.

The following year, in 1929, Martínez expresses his concern with poor maternal-infant health in his province, which had been uncovered by some research his office had undertaken: "Ambato, in relation to the number of its inhabitants, is at the head of the cities that have the highest percentage of still births [*nacido-muertos*]. In addition, the mortality rate of infants under one year of age and of women from puerperal infection is also among the highest. This is because 90 percent of women are attended in births by empiric hands [untrained midwives] and in the worst hygienic conditions. Infant feeding is also devoid of any scientific principles and the care and cleanliness of it is almost zero."[13] The identification of this problem arose through the process of collection and analysis of statistics, which was an important part of Sanidad work. (The fact that the Sanidad undertook collection and analysis of information to develop its priorities for intervention did not prevent it from building in a series of assumptions about who was responsible for health problems, such as blaming mothers for their children's poor health.[14]) Like others in the Sanidad, Martínez also contextualized his jurisdiction within a comparative context, which helped him to assess which areas should be prioritized for urgent attention. Given that the Asistencia Pública had access to more funds (drawing on rental income from the institution's large rural properties), the Sanidad delegate urged the Asistencia agency to invest some of their resources in adapting a room to establish a small maternity service in the provincial hospital. "I believe that there could be no better investment of this money than what I request, which would save many mothers and children and would be a true school of hygiene for a good portion of the population." It was difficult to believe, he commented, that the province did not yet have such a service. Unfortunately, Martínez felt compelled to circumvent the provincial subdirector of Asistencia Pública and to write directly to the director of Asistencia Pública in Quito with this suggestion, because "motives of personal enmity would cause my petition to be rejected by the Sr. Subdirector of Asistencia Pública, thus I find myself in the position of having to direct myself to you." Strained relations were interfering with Martínez's ability to advance evidence-based projects to address important health problems.

In Ambato as elsewhere in Ecuador, given the Asistencia Pública's overall responsibility for curative facilities such as hospitals, this agency provided the supplies in the isolation wards while the Sanidad offered the medical staff who attended patients there with infectious diseases. Shortly after the discussion of birthing conditions, the tension between the Asistencia Pública and the Sanidad in Ambato further deepened when Martínez was infected with typhoid fever in the hospital. Martínez attributed his illness to the lack of basic supplies provided by the Asistencia Pública in their management of the hospital.

> Without doubt the costly illness that I have just experienced, and from which I am still recuperating, was contracted in the Hospital; there were innumerable times that I had to leave after a hospital visit without disinfecting my hands, to avoid conflicts that arise over a capsule of sublimate [*pastilla de sublimado*] or a small amount of alcohol for disinfection. The situation of the Isolation Ward has been so deplorable, that it seems incredible that I have had to obligate family members of patients to provide soap to wash clothes, water, fruit juices, medications and even food; for all of these supplies are denied to us, systematically.[15]

He pointed out that under the law, it was the Asistencia Pública that was responsible for the care of patients, not the Sanidad, and therefore he requested that the isolation ward be turned over to the Asistencia

Pública's care before his medical leave ended and he returned to work. "The spirit of sacrifice that any Physician must have obligates me to continue attending at the Hospital, but there is no moral or human law that compels me to sacrifice my Señora and four little children by exposing them to diseases, as necessarily would happen, considering the nonexistent protection that exists in the Establishment."

While the director general of Sanidad, by then Dr. Alfonso Mosquera Narváez, understood the delegate's reasoning, he felt it was essential that Sanidad physicians retain control of the ward due to the nature of the diseases treated there. He did pass on to his counterpart at the head of the Asistencia Pública agency the commentary about the hospital conditions.[16] That official, Augusto Egas, agreed with the characterization of the locale of the isolation ward, confirming that it was "narrow, unhygienic, without separation; it is imperative that it receive immediate attention."[17] Not surprisingly, in the response of Ambato's subdirector of Asistencia Pública that Egas transcribed within his message to Mosquera Narváez, Dr. Rafael A. Sevilla denied all of Martínez's accusations. Indeed, he went so far as to speculate that the typhoid fever had originated in Martínez's home and that he had been the one who had introduced it into the hospital. Given this ongoing conflict, Egas suggested that it would be opportune if he and Mosquera Narváez could travel together to Ambato to try to resolve the situation. In the meantime, Martínez had already gone over Mosquera Narváez's head by sending his petition to be excused from attending patients with infecto-contagious diseases in the isolation ward to the minister of social welfare.[18] Mosquera Narváez again insisted on the Sanidad retaining control of this service. On the same day, he heard from Egas that Sevilla had informed him that Asistencia Pública physicians had been attending patients in the isolation ward for several weeks, and that they would prefer to continue to do so.[19] Perhaps the Asistencia continued to treat those patients, or maybe Egas and Mosquera Narváez did go to Ambato to mediate this dispute, as it subsides from the archival documentation. Any resolution seems to have depended on the good relationship between Egas and Mosquera Narváez and their joint commitment to resolve the dispute and find a solution palatable to both local officials.

Another fraught relationship was between the Sanidad delegation and the municipality, given that the latter was responsible for a suite of health-related activities and infrastructure: garbage collection, inspection of markets, installation of potable water and drainage systems, and so on. Tension with the municipal physician was alluded to in Suárez's February 1927 comments about the physician's lack of communication and coordination with the delegate. In mid-January 1929, Martínez presented his annual address about the hygiene projects the municipality should undertake in the coming year to a session of the Ambato municipal council. He started by pointing out that he was fulfilling his duty to provide these instructions under Article 14 of the Ley de Sanidad. He then comments, "It doesn't matter if this report is filed away, without the municipal government even seeing it, as occurred last year; in submitting it I am simply complying with a legal obligation, and the desire to see Ambato benefit from Hygiene projects."[20] It is difficult to overlook the frustrated tone of this introduction, suggesting ongoing tensions, which itself may have made the council disinclined to consider his recommendations. In general, archival documents suggest that the relations between municipal councils and the public health service had been difficult for the previous fifteen years, as chapter 2 indicates. By the mid-1920s these relations had become sufficiently fraught that the renewed Conservative Party had identified municipal autonomy as a central piece of its party platform, one facet of a general position favoring local autonomy over the state expansionism that was a hallmark of the Juliana governments.[21] Without doubt, relations between municipal governments and central state agencies needed to be managed with considerable diplomacy. In his report, Martínez then went on to enumerate the many deficiencies of the municipal services provided and the need for investment of significantly more resources in improving these services to meet the municipality's obligations.

Even within the provincial Sanidad office itself, there were tensions. In 1935 a new outreach program for maternal-infant health was established by the national service,[22] redefining this area of care as a preventive health issue, thus falling under the Sanidad's mandate. University-trained midwives and nurses were appointed to each provincial public health delegation to provide free obstetrical and neonatal services to women with limited resources in provincial cities and a few cantonal seats (*cabeceras de cantón*) but not primarily in rural areas. Sanidad-employed midwives were authorized to run a parallel private practice for patients able to pay for their services. Early on, Martínez was pleased with the professionalism of newly appointed state midwife Consuelo Rueda in 1936 and compared her favorably to the first person employed briefly in this role. Before long, however, this relationship also deteriorated. In early 1937, Martínez accused Rueda of having signed birth certificates for deliveries attended by one of Ambato's unlicensed (or empiric) midwives, Rosa de Gómez. Rueda admitted to the regional director of Sanidad in Quito that she had done so but explained that it was in response to "pleas and tears from those who thus save themselves from paying a fine and other difficulties." She had agreed to do this as a kind of interim measure, she said, just "until the people become moralized and accustomed to the idea that without the certificate of a professional there will be no registration [of a birth in the civil registry], and thus they will seek out only professionals and not empirics."[23] It is possible that, given Rueda's positioning as someone without local social networks, she necessarily relied on compromises with other local practitioners and an understanding of the broader dilemmas facing her potential clients in order to bring people into the maternal-infant health program. This pragmatic attitude was contrary to how Martínez had advertised this new maternal-infant health service in a flyer his office produced when the program was inaugurated. There he insisted on a much more rigid approach, communicating to local residents that "with the availability of free services of a professional, there is no reason to expose yourself to the dangers of empirics, to whom we will apply the sanction established in Article 56.4 of the Public Health Police Code (Código de Policía Sanitaria), if they continue to illegally exercise the profession of midwifery."[24] While Martínez requested Rueda be fired,[25] the regional subdirector of Sanidad in Quito seemed to hold a different view of the seriousness of her contravention. Indeed, her adaptations to the local conditions may have helped her gain clients for the program, which successfully increased the number of births in the area that occurred with some kind of professional attention.[26] Soon thereafter, Rueda stopped reporting to the provincial delegate and began to send her monthly reports directly to Sanidad officials in Quito instead, which appears to be both an expression of her difficult relationship with Martínez and an acknowledgment of the value of her work in the eyes of more distant Sanidad leaders.

Rueda wasn't the only subordinate colleague with whom Martínez was displeased. One of the first Sanidad nurses appointed to this program in Ambato was accused by the delegate of "seeming to be dedicated more to prostitution than to fulfilling her noble mission."[27] In speculating about why Consuelo Rueda in turn did not meet his expectations, he suggested at one point that her poor work might be due to her "habitual alcoholism."[28] The weight of archival evidence shows considerable competence of the female employees working in this program, and also shows an uncomfortable relationship in many cases between these female professionals and their higher-ranking male supervisors, who seemed nonplussed by working with independent professional women who generally were unmarried, were not from the local area, and had a less elite background than physicians. The conflicts in Ambato appear at one pole of a general tendency toward tensions between female Sanidad practitioners and their male physician supervisors, laden with hierarchies among medical fields as well as with gendered and class dimensions.

Persuasively, in response to the delegate's ongoing criticisms, Rueda defended herself in September 1940 by pointing out that in four and a half years in Ambato she had not had a single case of puerperal infection, much less a death under her care.[29] While there were some public complaints against her during her tenure in Ambato, they were limited to her occasional unavailability and to the fact that she did not provide all supplies. However, her understanding was that clients were perfectly satisfied with her services until they arrived at the provincial Sanidad delegation to obtain a birth certificate and were subjected to an interrogation to discover whether the midwife had provided all of the necessary supplies at no cost. While the program aspired to provide supplies for births, none of the state midwives in this program regularly received the supplies that were supposed to be provided to them by regional Sanidad offices. In some cases, Rueda was even formally fined by the police, apparently at the delegate's instigation, for not being available to attend all patients who sought her services, which left little of her salary for her living expenses. But as she explained, "It is impossible to attend to everyone, because often I am away on extended calls, and so of course, I am not at home when they come looking for my services."[30] Indeed, in the month to which she referred in this note, she had delivered nineteen babies, almost twice the minimum expectations for midwives in these positions (who regularly also provided many dozens of prenatal consultations in a month). It is interesting to consider whether her difficult relationship with her supervisor, which was made visible to some of her clients, may have positively impacted her reputation in Ambato among some sectors.

Underlying much of the Sanidad's work is a deepening process of recognition—an implicit acknowledgment of the agency's legitimacy in undertaking their programs, a legitimacy that was painstakingly built across many relationships and domains. What is revealed by a case where the ordinary routines of state activity do not work smoothly? Where a government office faces problems of recognition? The point here is not that the Tungurahua Sanidad office had no successes—it did. Rather, this case helps us identify some of the difficulties, structural as well as more personal, that public health officials had to confront. Was the situation in Ambato due to idiosyncrasies—just a reflection of Martínez's temperament? Or was there a deeper difficulty related to the immersion in local relations that made some of these relationships more fraught than when a higher or more distant authority expressed his opinion? What was the optimal balance between familiarity with local social relations and enough distance to seem to stand above them, as Sanidad officials so often aspired to do?

These materials also underline how important what we would now call "soft skills" were in the work the Sanidad was undertaking. For a physician in general, excellent technical skills had to be combined with good "bedside manner" and communication with patients. In private practice, many of Martínez's demanding standards would have made him an excellent clinician—it would have been only to himself that he would have been applying that exacting standard of care. Spending over a decade and a half as delegate of Sanidad may not have made the best use of his skills, given what appears to have been a rather prickly temperament when it came to relations with colleagues.

And it cannot have been easy to find a candidate better suited to the particular demands of this position, given the few physicians in the province and the oft-lamented "urbanismo" that drew these practitioners to the country's largest urban centers. An additional complication was the low salaries in Ambato of the provincial delegate and other Sanidad employees, something that Martínez pointed out several times in the late 1930s. For instance, in 1940 the salary of the delegate had been frozen for the previous ten years, resulting in a monthly pay of only 250 sucres, while the three municipal physicians in the province's other cantons earned twice that at 500 sucres.[31] It wasn't only his own salary that concerned him: the office clerk—a white-collar employee who did important work managing the documentation and production of statistics that was central to Sanidad activities—only earned 100 sucres per month, less than a bricklayer or carpenter as Martínez pointed out.[32] In Martínez's opinion, inadequate remuneration had an impact on how the public viewed Sanidad officials: "Under these conditions our prestige as professionals is undermined, since the public assumes that only physicians with little preparation would accept such a poorly remunerated position."[33] This situation may have made it difficult for him to have the appropriate legitimacy to exercise leadership over both the municipal physicians and the Asistencia Pública physicians in the ways that the law set out, leaving him in an awkward position to navigate his relationship with colleagues in other institutions.

These factors seem to have been markedly more problematic in the small professional circles of a provincial city like Ambato than in a larger milieu like Quito. For context, to Tungurahua province's 20 physicians in 1941, Pichincha province where Quito was located had 168, while Guayas province centered on Guayaquil had 189. Their population counts did not merit this vast difference. In 1942, the provincial population was estimated at 207,138 for Tungurahua, 305,175 for Pichincha, and 415,734 for Guayas.[34] In other words, Tungurahua had about two-thirds the population of Pichincha, but only 12 percent of the physicians

Table 4.1. Professionals in Ecuador in 1941

Province	Physician	Dentist	Optician	Midwife	Vet
Highlands					
Imbabura	17	5		4	
Pichincha	168	36	2	8	10
Cotopaxi	15	4			
Tungurahua	20	5		1	1
Chimborazo	20	6		2	
Bolívar	10	1			
Cañar	5	1			
Azuay	47	8			2
Loja	16	5		3	
Coast					
El Oro	5	4			
Guayas	189	47		17	1
Los Ríos	7	2	1		
Manabí	30	8			
Esmeraldas	5	1			1

Province	Engineer	Architect	Lawyer	Accountant
Highlands				
Imbabura	4		12	6
Pichincha	77	17	180	91
Cotopaxi	6		13	1
Tungurahua	5		18	8
Chimborazo	5		19	10
Bolívar	1		9	2
Cañar			15	3
Azuay	7		90	13
Loja	7		42	3
Coast				
El Oro	1		7	3
Guayas	32	7	107	133
Los Ríos			9	12
Manabí	5	1	23	17
Esmeraldas	2		3	8

***Source*: Dirección Nacional de Estadística, *Ecuador en cifras*, 113.**

of the latter. Most other provincial contexts were similar to Tungurahua in this regard, vividly demonstrating the allure of the country's two or three main cities for physicians. The distribution of different kinds of professionals[35] (see table 4.1) across Ecuador's provinces in 1941 (with the exception of the Amazon region, the Galápagos Islands, and the northernmost province of Carchi) displays clearly the concentration of professionals in Pichincha and Guayas, followed by Azuay province, the location of Ecuador's third largest city, Cuenca.

There also seem to have been fewer situations where people would seek out the Sanidad delegation in Tungurahua to help them resolve problems. Perhaps the poorer mediation skills of Martínez—and the lesser legitimacy that he feared arose from his low salary—removed him from such a role. When the public did approach the Sanidad, it was more likely with a subordinate employee such as Consuelo Rueda, and the fact that she was disciplined by Martínez for taking a more flexible approach and engaging in compromises that could both benefit members of the public and enhance her own acceptance among them highlights Martínez's divergent view of how the Sanidad should achieve its goals. He didn't seem to see his role in the way several other successful public health leaders did, where their skills in mediation were so important to their activities. Rather, he emphasized more his goals of raising the standards of public health, standards that he frequently pointed out to colleagues when he felt that they had failed to achieve them. Paradoxically, this seems to have made it more difficult for him to stand apart from and above local social relations, and thus to contribute to the reification of the state that often seemed to result from everyday public health encounters.

In addition to being well-trained physicians, public health leaders developed a broader vision that came from their work for an institution of national scope. Local ways of doing things were compared with and brought into alignment with best practices from elsewhere. The implications of local practices could impact other regions if a disease outbreak was not effectively managed: this could be urgent for a location like Ambato, which had been a significant outbreak location for plague. However, there is no single typical case that can serve as a microcosm of the whole—each location had its own unique set of challenges and opportunities as well as particular configuration of local social relations and histories, as we also saw in the plague outbreaks in Alausí and Guaytacama. Different alignments of local and more distant social actors enabled or constrained Sanidad activities within what were always specifically situated—and never generic—regional spaces.

Chapter 5

Regulating Pharmacies and Professional Defense in Highland Ecuador

Shortly after the creation of the subdirectorate of Sanidad in Quito in early 1914, its officials informed the Quito police that there were many *empíricos* (empirics, or unlicensed practitioners) who treated and prescribed drugs for the city's poor population. They constituted a "social plague" for medicine, just as *tinterillos* (informal lawyers or scribes) did for law, and therefore the authorities should act to prevent the increase in *curanderos* (healers) who lacked entirely any kind of scientific knowledge. In order to achieve this goal, the subdirector asked the police intendant to prohibit the owners of pharmacies from filling prescriptions that were not signed by physicians as well as to prevent pharmacists from themselves prescribing medications, since they might do so with the sole purpose of profiting from filling such prescriptions.[1]

Prior to the passage of the Ley de Boticas y Droguerías, or Law of Pharmacies, in November 1920 (and its associated Reglamento—the regulation by means of which it was implemented—in February 1921), the role of the Sanidad in monitoring pharmacies was poorly defined. If there were irregularities at pharmacies, it was primarily the dean of the Faculty of Medicine at the Universidad Central who was empowered to order inspections of pharmacies.[2] However, the Reglamento de Boticas y Droguerías of 1921 changed that, stating squarely in its first article that "the exercise of the pharmacy profession, the sale of drugs and medicinal preparations, the preparation and sale of pharmaceutical specialties, of chemical products, serums, vaccine, antitoxins and opotherapeutic preparations, are under the authority and jurisdiction of the Public Health Service (Servicio de Sanidad Pública), which will have under its responsibility the monitoring and compliance with the Ley de Boticas y Droguerías and this Regulation." This legislation brought yet another area of health-related practices under the umbrella of Sanidad work and opens up additional opportunities for analysis of the agency's varied roles that together helped conjure the state.

Along with overseeing pharmacies, the monitoring of licensed and unlicensed medical practitioners—activities that were labeled "professional defense" in Ecuador—came under the responsibility of the Sanidad service in the 1920 Ley, which brought the Universidad Central into dialogue with the Sanidad in a variety of contexts discussed below. The dispensing of drugs held a central place in the constellation of issues involving regulation of medical professionals. During the first two decades of the Ley's application, the interests of different groups—physicians, medical students, graduated pharmacists, pharmacy students, owners of small and large pharmacies, and unlicensed dispensers—became aligned or conflicted with each other in a range of ways in relation to three key spheres of activity: the prescribing of drugs, the preparation of drugs, and the sale of drugs. These were all areas where various groups vied over who should be authorized to carry out these activities and who had the right to monitor them. Differing dimensions of Sanidad work intersected here: regulation of commerce and of product quality, regulation of professions and credentials, and compliance with international agreements regarding opiates, among others. While there were a number of ways that the Sanidad intervened in other commercial issues—such as monitoring the hygienic preparation and sale of food items and ensuring the quality of milk (by overseeing municipal work in these areas)—these came together in a distinctive and more direct way in the regulation of pharmacies. While in some ways the political instability of the 1930s generated obstacles in the smooth functioning of this system, it also stimulated intensified lobbying by various groups to pursue their interests, all of which enabled new forms of negotiation by the Sanidad. In this, as in other areas under its mandate, the Sanidad worked to set itself apart from and above the stakeholder groups to act as a mediator of their interests.

While the 1914 incident that opens this chapter suggests that alternative healers posed a danger, the archival record shows much greater concern over partially trained biomedical practitioners than with people working within a substantially different healing tradition who did not prescribe drugs. This highlights the pivotal role of pharmacies for regulating medicine that involved drug therapies and also may suggest that there were simply fewer strategic sites where the state could monitor other forms of healing. The Sanidad did, however, monitor ambulant sales of medicinal products, which occurred in very visible places in urban streets and plazas.

Diagnosing Illness and Prescribing Treatments

In Ecuador, a range of people participated in diagnosing illness and prescribing treatments (including medications): not only physicians but also medical students whose studies were not yet complete, other kinds of healers, and indeed, pharmacists themselves. As I have argued elsewhere regarding both obstetrical care and nursing,[3] licensed healthcare providers existed within a larger ecosystem of practitioners with whom they sometimes competed.[4] With the passage of the 1920 Ley de Boticas, graduated and licensed physicians were clearly defined as those authorized to prescribe drug therapies. Even so, this authorization was not without its exceptions: in smaller population centers, the Sanidad could formally approve other practitioners—and sometimes even recruited their help in public health outreach campaigns—provided that there were no physicians in the area. Once licensed practitioners set up practice in such locations, however, they could activate the Ley's provisions to close down other practices via the mechanism of petitioning the Sanidad to prohibit unlicensed practitioners, orders that could trigger penalties if they were ignored. This was akin to some other entitlements that required people to take the initiative to claim their rights through petitioning state agents, foregrounding such officials' roles in interceding and mediating among members of the population.

The ability to prescribe drugs was a key node in professional defense processes. The Sanidad kept a registry (*nómina*) of licensed practitioners and in the 1920s began to provide such lists formally to pharmacies to ensure that pharmacists would not fill prescriptions written by unlicensed practitioners.[5] Creating the nómina[6] also required that all graduated physicians register their academic credentials with the Sanidad, although it was the Universidad Central (yet another institution with which the Sanidad was in tension) rather than the Sanidad that determined what constituted those credentials. Among the legislated measures that the subdirector of Sanidad underlined for the pharmacists of the capital in May 1921 was the provision that it was absolutely prohibited to fill prescriptions written by empirics or medical students.[7] Of course, the existence of such a law did not on its own ensure that it was followed. In November 1924, the Sanidad's Comisión Inspectora de Boticas (Pharmacy Inspection Commission) felt the need to remind all of Quito's pharmacy owners and the pharmacists they employed that the Ley and Reglamento "prohibit dispatching without a physician's prescription [*receta*] those medications that are not in constant use in domestic Medicine and that due to their inoffensive nature, physicians often prescribe verbally."[8]

To further strengthen the implementation of the Sanidad's registry, pharmacists were required to establish within each pharmacy their own registry of the signatures of all licensed physicians who were in practice in Quito. An additional dimension of monitoring physicians' activities was also put in place, with the requirement that each pharmacy report monthly to the Sanidad the details of which physicians had prescribed medications that had opiates as an ingredient and in what amounts. This served a dual function, as it provided an opportunity to identify specific physicians who might be overprescribing (and possibly enabling the consumption habits of a small number of known illicit drug users in Quito) at the same time as it permitted compliance with the government's reporting requirements under international agreements dealing with what were called heroic drugs.

Both physicians and pharmacies therefore were subject to new forms of oversight, while simultaneously they received enhanced forms of protection of their professional rights under this legislation. This was a common trade-off of new rights and new responsibilities as Sanidad activities expanded. Even when it came to registering their credentials, however, not all physicians were willing to recognize the right of the Sanidad to participate in regulating them when this was first instituted.[9] This is reminiscent of the Sanidad's struggle to persuade physicians to disclose incidents of infecto-contagious diseases among their patients (see chapter 2), where doctors' failure to comply in both cases initially suggested an unwillingness to acknowledge the legitimacy of Sanidad oversight.

Two incidents in the 1920s show the connection between regulating pharmacies, on the one hand, and professional defense of physicians and monitoring of health workers, on the other. Soon after the passage of the 1920 Ley de Boticas, it was discovered that a medical student who had not yet completed his coursework had been treating a family among whom one member died from, and several others were infected with, typhoid fever. Physicians were required to report cases of infecto-contagious diseases to the Sanidad service so that it could devise measures to prevent their further spread. The student had not reported these cases and, in fact, claimed that his patient had died of other causes, despite the contrary reports of several experienced hospital and public health physicians. The student was deemed guilty of illegally exercising the medical profession, evidenced specifically by the fact that he was "prescribing medication all over the place" (*anda recetando por todas partes*).[10] The next month the Facultad de Medicina, Cirugía y Farmacia denounced that they were aware of numerous medical students who similarly "exercise publicly the medical profession and as a result prescribe medication, prescriptions that are filled in the pharmacies and drugstores of the city without hesitation."[11] The Faculty of Medicine that was at such pains to prevent the premature exercise of the medical profession by their students would however put just as much energy into defending their exclusive right to practice once they had graduated.

This same suite of provisions could be activated against another category of practitioners, as a 1926 case demonstrates. The midwife Carmela Granja was Quito's most notorious (and sought after) abortionist.[12] Like the 1921 medical student, she was trained in the biomedical model at the Universidad Central, having undertaken all four years of the Facultad de Medicina's midwifery training program, although she was expelled in 1920 before graduating (possibly it was discovered that she had already begun to offer abortions). Without formal credentials, she nonetheless operated a busy obstetrical clinic in Quito from the 1920s on, although her practice was interrupted by several conflicts with the Sanidad and the police and at least two jail terms in the 1930s. In September 1926, she was called to the offices of the Sanidad to answer for her illegal exercise of a profession, since she was offering obstetrical services without having graduated from the midwifery program at the university. While there was no mention there of abortions, on the same day, all pharmacists and pharmacy owners in Quito were reminded by the Sanidad of the absolute ban on accepting any prescriptions signed by midwives that contained "rue, savin, mugwort, saffron, rye ergot and other similar substances known as abortifacients."[13] The Sanidad may have had to fall back on the professional defense provisions due to a lack of sufficient evidence to charge her criminally for offering abortions, but the memo to the pharmacies demonstrates the mechanisms available in the Ley de Boticas to address their concerns.

Legal provisions of this kind also affected foreign physicians who sought to establish medical practices in Ecuador. Potentially they would pose greater competition to Ecuadorian physicians than practitioners with less formal training, since they would be more likely to attract the same kinds of clients. For instance, in 1927, following a complaint to him by the Universidad Central, director general Pablo Arturo Suárez had to remind Sr. J. Mackensie (he pointedly did not refer to him as "Dr.") that the Código de Policía Sanitaria prohibited anyone from practicing a medical profession without having their academic degree approved by the Faculty of Medicine at the Universidad Central and then registered with the directorate of Sanidad.[14] In the late 1930s, an increasing number of foreign-trained physicians and other professionals migrated to Ecuador fleeing conflict in Europe, which made these cases more frequent. Ecuador was not unusual in requiring foreign-trained professionals to revalidate their credentials before initiating practice.

Medical consultation might also occur within pharmacies, and some accusations of *empiricismo* therefore relate to pharmacists and other pharmacy employees providing diagnostic and therapeutic suggestions to customers. The law worked to define more clearly the scope of physicians' and pharmacists' different rights and responsibilities, within a context in which medicine was dominant over pharmacy. One way that this hierarchy manifested itself was that while pharmacists could not diagnose illnesses and prescribe treatments, physicians could take on pharmacist roles, provided they were not also practicing medicine.[15] This was more likely to occur in provincial cities than in Quito, since there was more often a shortage of graduated pharmacists in provincial contexts. Another manifestation was that while pharmacists were empowered to question physicians' prescriptions, they were not authorized to change them. Moreover, within the Sanidad service, for many years it was a physician who headed up the Jefatura de Farmacias y Profesiones Médicas, thus taking the lead on monitoring pharmacies and pharmacists. It was only in the mid-1940s—about a quarter century after these activities began—that a pharmacist was named chief of this section of the Sanidad office.

In general, while there were clear spatial differences in how these regulations operated—with considerably more need for and tolerance of practitioners with less specialized training outside of Ecuador's largest cities—there were no doubt also class differences in how people sought treatment and remedies regardless of location. Wealthier patients were in a position to be attended by physicians and purchase medications at formal pharmacies, while those with fewer resources were likely treated more informally in small-scale venues known as *botiquines*.

Preparing and Dispensing Drugs

The 1920 Ley and 1921 Reglamento not only defined who could prescribe drug therapies but also identified who could prepare and dispense drugs—specifically, graduated pharmacists. Even so, the archival record prompts the question, which pharmacists? If a graduated pharmacist owned a pharmacy, he (they were mostly men) couldn't also practice as a pharmacist: the professional responsibilities of pharmacists and pharmacy owners were not the same and could potentially be in conflict. And in turn, if a pharmacist had credentials as both a physician and a pharmacist, he could only practice one of those professions. These provisions aimed to eliminate conflicts of interest and maintain checks and balances, so that profit-making motives would not contaminate professional judgments about appropriate treatments (as suggested by the 1914 concerns of the Sanidad that open this chapter).

These restrictions could generate staffing shortages in smaller population centers: for instance, in Ibarra, capital of Imbabura province north of Pichincha, there were some graduated pharmacists who were not practicing their profession (whether because they were busy administering family agricultural estates or employed to teach science in the state high school), others who were also physicians, and others who owned pharmacies. Very few remained who had the time, or were legally in a position, to exercise their profession. This led the Sanidad to authorize some other experienced but unlicensed practitioners—called *practicantes*—to dispense drugs. After 1920 there was an increasing formalization of the qualifications that practicantes had to present in order to obtain permission to practice, eventually culminating in 1939 in the establishment of formal *cursos de capacitación* (training courses). Practicantes fell into two categories: those who worked in pharmacies owned by others and those who had experience in such work and wished to set up their own botiquines. Again, in smaller population centers such as cantonal seats (*cabeceras de cantón*) where there were no licensed pharmacists, the law allowed practicantes to set up commercial venues where medications were sold, provided they were approved by the provincial Sanidad delegate, who played a key role in managing these permissions.

Graduated pharmacists behaved as a group in several ways. They formed a network through their experience of studying at one of the main universities in the country. In Quito and the north central highlands, most graduated pharmacists had studied at the Universidad Central, and the archives showed that the university continued to advocate for them after they completed their studies. In Quito, they were also organized in a professional association, the Asociación de Farmacéuticos de Quito. Pharmacists organized collectively to have their expertise recognized and to protect their professional space: most importantly, their sole right to produce complex pharmaceutical preparations, known as *recetas magisteriales*.

A significant resource at their disposal was the law itself. The first article of the 1920 Ley stated unequivocally that every pharmacy must be under the direct supervision of a pharmacist and that only in these establishments was it permitted to dispatch prescriptions or sell medications, except for the sale of everyday domestic remedies as determined in the regulation. However, the low number of graduated pharmacists made it difficult to enforce this provision strictly. The Reglamento formally recognized this reality and institutionalized the unevenness over space that was so common with issues of this kind. Article 3 specified that where there was no graduated pharmacist available, a physician could oversee a pharmacy, provided that he wasn't also exercising the medical profession. And if there was no physician available, then the Sanidad could authorize another person to run a pharmacy, "as long as they can demonstrate general knowledge and experience in the preparation and sale of medications for a period of no less than four years." In either case, however, this permission would expire one year after a pharmacy was established in that location under the direction of a licensed pharmacist. Wherever possible—which was only in large cities where there were sufficient professionals—the Reglamento also mandated that in each pharmacy there should be both a principal pharmacist (*farmacéutico principal*) and a substitute pharmacist (*regente sustituto*) who would assume responsibility for the pharmacy during hours and days when the principal was absent and especially in evenings when they were *de turno* (alternating shifts when different pharmacies were assigned the responsibility to stay open to serve the public). In addition, the Reglamento provided that no one with another job incompatible with his or her presence in the pharmacy could serve as principal pharmacist nor could a pharmacist direct more than one pharmacy at a time. In addition to the division of labor to avoid conflicts of interest, this also points to the necessity of having a pharmacist available to serve clients and oversee preparation of medication on a continuous basis.

These provisions outlined a best-case scenario and often weren't practical. Shortages of licensed pharmacists were sufficiently persistent to require formal amendments to the Ley de Boticas. For instance, in 1937 an addition to the law specified that, despite the general rules, when a location had fewer than one pharmacy run by a licensed pharmacist for each five thousand inhabitants, the regional Sanidad office could authorize the operation of pharmacies "represented by persons who demonstrate [*acrediten*] having general knowledge of Pharmacy and no less than 15 years of practice in the preparation of medications, to the satisfaction of the Director of Sanidad of the respective Zone and by means of a test of aptitude [*prueba de aptitud*], rendered before a Commission designated by the General Directorate of Sanidad."[16] The clause also added that, again under authorization from the directorate, graduated chemists could also run (*regentar*) pharmacies.

Archival sources demonstrate that there were various ways that pharmacists mobilized collectively to defend their professional rights. Sometimes, university officials led the charge in their defense. In 1929, the dean of the Facultad de Medicina denounced the infringement of the Ley de Boticas by various pharmacy owners who employed empíricos to fill prescriptions.[17] The claim was couched in terms, first, of the "elementary principle of morality and social security" and, second, of professional defense: "The Law has established, quite rightly, that only professionals can attend to physicians for their prescriptions and remedies, for security and in protection of the lives of the public." This followed a similar complaint by Francisco J. Barba in the Sindicato Médico, an association of physicians,[18] which prompted the director of Sanidad to appoint a commission to investigate.

The following year, in 1930, representatives of the Asociación de Farmacéuticos de Quito, led by José Camilo Pacheco, Juan Escalante Pino, and J. Aurelio Miño, launched something of a campaign in defense of their professional jurisdiction. They petitioned the minister of social welfare and labor directly, explaining that the law required that a graduated pharmacist oversee any dispensing of drugs, not only in privately owned pharmacies but also in health care facilities (hospitals, social welfare institutions, and private clinics). Their main complaint was that the drug repository (*gran droguería*) of the Asistencia Pública was directed by the Hermanas de la Caridad (Sisters of Charity religious order), as were the dispensaries (*boticas*) of the Hospital Civil and the Hospital Militar.[19] The pharmacists asked the minister to take appropriate action "in order to avoid infringement of the Law, trampling our rights, which we know how to defend very decidedly, under the protection of your wise measures, which will also benefit the remedy-seeking public and even hospital patients."[20]

The minister passed on this complaint to the director general of Sanidad, who investigated. His response reveals a gendered dimension to the issue of professional credentials as well as provides insight into the medication supply chain. The director general explained that the facility that the Asistencia Pública managed was not a commercial pharmacy but rather a drug repository.[21] It supplied medications to its own healthcare institutions, which were administered by the Hermanas de la Caridad.[22] Because the Junta Central de Asistencia Pública was the government agency authorized to import narcotics, it also supplied the various private pharmacies of Quito with these medications. In other words, the Hermanas did not fill prescriptions but instead supplied the raw materials that were used by licensed pharmacists to prepare medications in the pharmacies where they worked. The Botica del Hospital Civil San Juan de Dios, in turn, was directed by an Hermana whose credentials had been authorized by a decree in 1905, which had not been revoked.

Digging deeper, the records of the Universidad Central show that in 1905 and 1906, some nineteen nuns who had been serving as apothecaries in Ecuadorian health care institutions wrote examinations at the university to verify their knowledge of pharmacy practice, after which they were permitted to practice. Concurrent with the verification by the university of the Hermanas' practical knowledge of pharmacy, in 1904–

1905 a handful of young secular women took advantage of an opportunity to pursue a year of preparatory studies in 1904 and then four years of pharmacy studies. Special permission was required from the university rector to admit them, since they did not have the usual prerequisites for university study—hence also the need for a preparatory year. As secretary of education Luis A. Martínez describes this in his 1905 annual report: "In the past year on an experimental basis we established a basic course [*curso inferior*] in Pharmacy for señoritas. The initial results have surpassed all of the government's expectations."[23] A small cohort of four female students graduated from this pilot program in 1909.[24] When they completed their studies, they were considered "*licenciadas*" in pharmacy. While this term normally indicates completion of an undergraduate degree, it was later clarified that this literally meant that they were licensed to practice (although not to prepare more complex prescriptions) rather than had received the university degree known as a *licenciatura*. No more women were accepted to study pharmacy until the 1920s, when they began to be admitted with the same qualifications as men; the first woman graduated with a full pharmacy degree in 1929.[25]

Another group that took an active interest in whether pharmacies were employing sufficient numbers of licensed professionals was pharmacy students, especially as they approached graduation. They could be quite vocal in their campaign to secure positions in attractive locations like Quito (they would likely have been able to find work in smaller provincial cities, if they had been willing to move, given the shortages of pharmacists in those locations). They took it upon themselves, in 1932, to pass on information to the Sanidad about discussions within the Universidad Central's Pharmacy School, applauding the Sanidad's renewed emphasis on inspecting pharmacies. At their recent meeting, they explained, they had formally agreed to "applaud sincerely the attitude of the Commission and the Sr. Director, vanguard of professional defense. This observance of the law is of direct interest to us students of Pharmacy of the Central, who pledge to remain alert to the regeneration movement that has been launched against the antiscientific and illegal condescendence that until now Ecuadorian Pharmacy has suffered."[26] A year later, in February 1933, the university launched a broader campaign, with a formal request to the Sanidad by the rector of the university, who by then was former director general of Sanidad Suárez. Couching the concern in much broader language about the public interest and suggesting the university's desire to be more involved in monitoring the situation, he writes that the Faculty of Medicine "cannot remain indifferent in the face of the dangers to health and public well-being posed by the negligence of certain pharmacies, both in the Capital and in many provincial towns, in respect to personnel, material, implements and medications." He continues that the university was generally concerned to promote the interests of its graduates, and that "today, I refer specifically to the graduates of Pharmacy, who feel strongly injured in their rights and disappointed in their just aspirations, when they see that within Pharmacies it is common to employ an empiric instead of a professional."[27] He called on the director to work with the rector, the School of Pharmacy, the municipality, and the dean of medicine to collaborate in promoting pharmacists' interests.

Soon thereafter, in June and July 1933, there was a flurry of such lobbying activity by students, recently graduated pharmacists, and the university. Perhaps they identified a window of opportunity with the rapidly changing political terrain: there were three different ministers of government and social welfare in 1933 alone, tied to the frequent changes in the national presidency in the early 1930s. The intensity of activity suggests that there may have been a minister who they expected to be especially favorable to their position, or perhaps they simply took advantage of every available opportunity to present their claims. A new cycle of exchanges began in mid-June with a request from the minister of government and social welfare (no doubt prompted by a complaint to him) for a report from the director general of Sanidad about whether or not, in pharmacies in the provincial capitals, there were both principal and substitute pharmacists.[28] The director general explained that, given the shortage of pharmacists in provincial contexts, it was not practical to insist on having substitutes there. In Quito they could be stricter, but even so, pharmacy owners were still legally entitled to a grace period to give them time to replace pharmacists who had resigned from their positions. This had occurred recently, and the pharmacy owners had complied with the requirement to register this information with the Sanidad while they sought to hire replacements.[29] In the face of the minister's subsequent request for more information, the Sanidad produced two charts that demonstrated the agency's detailed attention to the pharmacy file. The charts included the list of all pharmacies and drugstores in the capital, their owners and their principal legal representatives (pharmacists), and "the complete list of the doctors of pharmacy and graduated pharmacists from the Universidad Central, whose total amounts to 55, of whom: 2 have died, 19 are absent from the city, 2 do not exercise the profession, 27 have other diverse occupations and 5 are available to be hired, the latter including 4 who have just recently graduated from the University."[30]

Even this wasn't sufficient information, however. The minister pointed out that the charts did not include substitute pharmacists. He recommended that at least those pharmacies of sufficient size to merit it be obligated to immediately contract substitutes, since he was aware of some graduated pharmacists available to fill these positions.[31] The director then communicated to all pharmacy owners in Quito about their obligation to appoint a substitute pharmacist. For good measure, he also published an announcement in the daily newspaper *El Comercio* calling all unemployed pharmacists to register their credentials and availability for employment in the Sanidad office. Without this information, it was difficult for the Sanidad to defend their professional rights. However, "unfortunately, only the Pharmacist Sr. Guillermo Arellano responded to our call, registering himself."[32] Since that same day the period conceded to the pharmacy owners to comply with the Sanidad order to appoint substitutes expired, and only four had obeyed the order, the director contacted the police intendant to seek the support of the *fuerza pública* (in the form of fifteen policemen) to back up the Sanidad comisario in closing down these businesses until they complied.

Additional information was then sent to the minister—a communication from the university rector and another from the Asamblea de Universidades—who passed it on to the Sanidad director. This included a list of five recent pharmacy graduates who were available for employment as principals as well as eight advanced pharmacy students who had completed their coursework and could serve as substitutes. The director general of Sanidad passed on the list of students to the pharmacy owners, with his authorization to employ them if graduated pharmacists were not available. Soon thereafter a meeting of pharmacists and pharmacy owners was convened with the minister, which resulted in an order to the Junta Central de Asistencia Pública to hire licensed pharmacists for their Almacén de Drogas and the Botica del Hospital.[33] This apparently didn't have any effect, however, since six months later the director asked the minister of government and Sanidad to resolve the ongoing issue of whether or not "it was possible to demand that the Junta Central de Asistencia Pública hire a pharmacist for their drug repository. On previous occasions when this same request has come from the unemployed pharmacists of this capital, my opinion together with that of the Sr. Director of Asistencia Pública, has been that for a simple drug repository, the Law and Regulation of Pharmacies does not apply."[34] Indeed, in 1936 a modification to the Law formally allowed the Hermanas de la Caridad to oversee specific pharmacies (within the hospitals they administered and in other establishments of Asistencia Pública or those run by the municipality), provided that they either could demonstrate that they had completed at least five years of satisfactory practice or had certificates confirming that they had studied pharmacy in an Ecuadorian university. This acknowledged and recognized the fact that in 1905 the Concejo Superior de Instrucción Pública had authorized their pharmacy work and subsequent governments had not rescinded that permission.

In November 1933, one of the more active recently graduated pharmacists, Colombian Braulio Montenegro, was still pressing these points in written requests to the Sanidad director. "As you know," he states,

> Currently in this capital there are several unemployed pharmacists. This is due to the fact that not all parts of the Ley de Boticas are implemented, requiring two pharmacists in each pharmacy, to ensure that the public is always attended by an expert [*técnico*]. Can you inform me why it is that all objections by these professionals have been denied? Currently in the Universidad Central there are seven pharmacy students completing their studies. This will cause a considerable increase in professional unemployment, so it is urgent that the Directorate of Sanidad take all pertinent measures. Otherwise, it is my belief that the School of Pharmacy should be closed, so that it does not uselessly produce professionals who will have no place to work.[35]

This flurry of activity—which could have significant outcomes, such as the closure of pharmacies—only showed one side of the picture, highlighting the activism and concerns of pharmacy graduates and students. The rather different perspective of pharmacy owners was expressed in response to these efforts, shedding light on the circumstances they faced. Elicio Flor, the owner of Quito's Botica Popular, provided a lengthy and detailed response to the Sanidad comisario's suggestion that he should employ two professional pharmacists. First, he pointed out that most pharmacies in Quito were small operations that generated a modest but decent living for their owners and could not possibly support the salaries of two pharmacists. These small establishments provided valuable services to the residents of Quito, but if they could not generate income for their owners, they would be destined to disappear. He then reflected that Ecuador suffered from the "superstition of the title," which led people to believe that only those with university degrees were competent, even though they might be unfit for a profession for other reasons. Civilized countries like England and Germany, he explained, were willing to accept certificates of aptitude and other evidence of experience and expertise in licensing professional practice. Following their model, if there was a person of well-known and long-term professional practice working in a pharmacy, there should be no need to have a substitute pharmacist on the payroll who would only upend the balance sheet of the small business. Drawing on all of these points, he argues:

> For my part I can and must say . . . that if I am obligated to pay another salary for a substitute pharmacist, I will find myself in the difficult situation of having to close down my business; and doubtless all of the other small pharmacy owners in Quito are in the same situation; and thus our constitutional right to freedom of work [*garantía constitucional de la libertad de trabajo*] will have been violated, because the truth is that what kind of liberty to work would there be if a business owner is obligated to pay expenses beyond the modest and usual profits of the enterprise? Not only will the right to work guaranteed by the Constitution perish, but also a large part of the industry itself will be destroyed to the detriment of the public, and all this just to secure impossible positions for a few unemployed professionals.

Finally, Flor pointed out that in his own case, he had more than fifty years of continuous practice in pharmacies in both the coastal region and the highlands. "What would someone like me do with a substitute pharmacist, in addition to the principal one that my pharmacy already has? He would be a supernumerary individual whose services are not needed by the pharmacy nor the public."[36] It seems that the vigorous insistence by the pharmacy students that they should have the sole right to practice when they completed their studies (or even before) exasperated this pharmacy owner sufficiently that he began to question the need for any formal training at all. The students were at risk of overplaying their hand.

Gathering and weighing the various and conflicting interests of the different stakeholder groups, the Sanidad proposed amending the regulation given that it had become impossible to apply due to both the scarcity of licensed pharmacists and the current economic situation, which was creating difficulties for many forms of commerce. The revisions created a new division of boticas in provincial capitals (including Quito, capital of Pichincha province as well as Ecuador's national capital) into first- and second-class establishments, authorizing the latter to have just one pharmacist instead of both a principal and a substitute. Where there were not sufficient licensed pharmacists, a practicante with ten years' experience could also be granted permission to serve as regente sustituto. In communicating the new classification via the four main newspapers in Quito, the resulting list indicated that there were only eight first-class pharmacies in the capital, while thirteen others were considered second class.[37] The category of "drugstore" (*droguería*) was also formalized for those venues where patent medicines were sold but medications were not actually prepared. This reclassification was certainly not the goal of the newly graduated pharmacists and university officials who initiated this discussion with their petitions and complaints: it reduced the positions for graduated pharmacists rather than increasing them. A process begun with one intention can (and often does) lead to an outcome neither anticipated nor desired by those who instigated it.

The level of political instability in the early 1930s had a marked impact on these processes. While there was considerable stability in the leadership of the Sanidad service—and therefore much longer institutional memory—the same cannot be said for the ministry that oversaw Sanidad. The fact that there were three different ministers just in 1933 seemed to encourage some groups to try again to get an advantageous answer from a new minister when they had failed with his predecessor. The director general of Sanidad alluded to this in a 1934 response where he felt he had to explain yet again the basic parameters of the situation and its recent history to a new appointee. The new minister had received a petition from a group of pharmacists. The director pointed out that there were no doubt files in the ministry archive about ongoing problems with the existing law governing pharmacies, which badly needed to be amended by Congress to meet more effectively the needs of the public, pharmacists, and pharmacy owners. At the same time, he explained, there had been a campaign by a few unemployed pharmacists who felt that the director general could and should provide them with work by obligating pharmacy owners to appoint both a principal and a substitute pharmacist. "Indeed, they have presented petitions to all of the Ministers who have held the portfolio of Government and Sanidad, all of them requesting, as they put it, that the Director of Sanidad fulfil his duty." Minister Manuel Balarezo, for instance, had been "caught unawares by a similar petition, whose result was that I had to order and carry out the closure of EIGHT PHARMACIES of this Capital, for not having two pharmacists in their employ. Naturally, this procedure raised a protest from the pharmacy owners, who *en masse* and with their respective lawyers, came to the Ministry to demand that the closure order be revoked." Once Balarezo heard their account, he canceled the closure order and approved instead modifications to the regulation to distinguish between first- and second-class pharmacies (as outlined above). Having done that, "of course these reforms were not to the liking of the unemployed pharmacists, since they did not offer them the positions that they were seeking." In response, they petitioned the subsequent minister, José Rafael Bustamente, and added to their request the in-house pharmacies of the hospitals and the *almacén de drogas* of the Junta Central de Asistencia Pública. It seems that they were unsuccessful with Bustamente, who ensured that the reformed regulation was implemented instead, to the dissatisfaction of the petitioners. "Given all of these antecedents and the terms of the current regulation, approved by your Ministry, it would not be appropriate to accept a new classification of the pharmacies that is proposed by the pharmacists who are signatories of the petition." Finally, the director also responded to the request that he provide access to his office's archives to the Sindicato de Farmacia so they could verify the work of the inspection commission that oversaw pharmacies. He was quite ready to do so, he said, if it were not that this group did not exist: "The so-called Sindicato de Farmacia is nothing of the kind, it is not a juridical entity, it has no legal representation, no one knows who its president is, nor where its meetings are held, the petition itself is signed illegibly by two beings called president and secretary of the session, etc., etc." In sum, he concluded that this petition was nothing more than another attempt by two or three unemployed pharmacists to coopt the authority of the director of Sanidad to obligate pharmacy owners, in contravention of the law, to employ them.[38] One outcome of these various petitions and activities in a context of rapidly changing personnel at the ministry was that the Sanidad took on the responsibility of sketching out the contours of the disputed terrain for the ministers as well as in mediating conflicts among the various parties. While political instability may have encouraged a flurry of lobbying activity, it also highlighted the greater knowledge Sanidad officials had of the ongoing issues and deeper context, such that political appointees might find they needed to depend on them more than would have occurred if they had time to settle into their roles.

The Sale of Drugs

A third activity in the constellation of dispensing of drugs was the sale of drugs. Some medications were highly controlled while others were considered "inoffensive" and therefore were easily accessible to consumers. According to the Law on Trade in Opium (Ley sobre el Comercio del Opio) of 1916, "commerce in unprocessed opium [*opio bruto*], medicinal opium and its alcaloides, salts and chemical derivatives, of cocaine and its salts, is reserved exclusively for owners of pharmacies and the directors of social welfare institutions."[39] This connected pharmacies (and the Sanidad) with issues of international trade in controlled substances. In response to consultations involving the chargé d'affaires of the British embassy, the minister of foreign relations, the dean of the Faculty of Medicine, and the Sanidad subdirector, the Ecuadorian president issued a clarifying executive decree in November 1922 indicating that pharmacy owners needed the authorization of the police chief (*intendente de policía*) to order from abroad any narcotic drugs, and on arrival, the customs authority would also review the documentation.[40] To streamline this process, in 1924 the importation of opium and similar heroic drugs

Table 5.1. Narcotics dispensed in Pichincha province, July 1922–June 1923

Drug	Amount (grams)
Opium	1,522
Morphine	250
Dionine	200
Codeine	178
Heroin	148
Cocaine	108
Novocain	12

***Source*: Data from Assistant physician of subdirectorate of Sanidad for Pichincha province to the minister of Sanidad, Quito, September 14, 1923, LCE-1923, ASS/MNM.**

was limited to the Juntas Centrales de Beneficencia de Quito, Guayaquil, and Cuenca, under the authorization of the ministry overseeing social welfare.[41] While this narrowed the route of importation (and likely simplified the process for pharmacies), pharmacy owners continued to be those exclusively authorized to sell the medicinal preparations made on-site by pharmacists with these raw ingredients.

In the 1920s and 1930s an escalating series of requirements were imposed on the owners of pharmacies. Ecuador's international treaties obligated the government to monitor and report on the sale of heroic substances such as morphine and opiates. In order for the Sanidad to compile, calculate, and pass on these figures, pharmacy owners were required to report on the exact amounts dispensed in their locales. For instance, the Sanidad was able to report to the minister the amounts of each such drug dispensed in medications in the province of Pichincha (primarily in Quito) during the twelve months from July 1922 to June 1923 (see table 5.1). In addition to helping the Sanidad meet international reporting requirements, collecting detailed data from each pharmacy and then bringing the figures together for the city and province provided a higher-level view revealing which specific physicians were prescribing these medications (something they might do in multiple pharmacies). This also allowed the Sanidad to monitor consumption patterns of a small number of known habitual users of these drugs. Again, by generating and compilating information from individual establishments, the Sanidad developed an overall understanding of the movement of narcotic medications that no individual pharmacy had.

In the context of the Sanidad's enhanced ability to monitor pharmacies and their products, correspondingly ambulant street vending of remedies was increasingly perceived as dangerous. An example of Sanidad reasoning appears in their response to a petition submitted to the minister of Sanidad to allow ambulant vending of medicinal products in September 1927. In his denial of this permit request, the Sanidad director outlined many objections to street vending of pharmaceutical products: the products usually contained an insufficient amount of the active ingredient; their price corresponded neither to the small amount of active ingredient nor to the value or volume of the inactive ingredient (most often soap, distilled water, or Vaseline); the claims about their effectiveness were overblown; and generally speaking, these sales lent themselves too easily to charlatanism.

> The buyer, in general, acquires these products casually, charmed by charlatanism, such that without any benefit whatsoever for the public, fabulous sales are made of these products. Completely susceptible, the passer-by purchases, for instance, a bar of soap that is famed to be a universal panacea, a soap that is neither really soap given the scarce quantity of the excipient [inactive substance], nor is it medicinal due to the scarce quantity of the active ingredient. The twenty cents that buyers pay in acquiring this unneeded product in a moment of suggestibility, don't even provide the benefit that a simple soap would offer, which at least would deliver cleanliness.[42]

The director of Sanidad pointed out that prohibiting these sales really functioned as a form of economic defense of the public under these circumstances. Framed as defense of the consumer, the underlying argument was that product quality was easier to monitor and ensure in licensed establishments—and indeed, the service spent a considerable amount of time inspecting pharmacies to verify that they stocked the appropriate list of items and that these were stored safely.

Increasingly drugs, vaccines, serums, and other pharmaceutical substances demanded more sophisticated storage conditions, such as refrigeration, in order to maintain their potency. This required pharmacy owners to make expensive investments in equipment. After 1920 there were also other minimum requirements that they had to meet in order to call their commercial establishments pharmacies, which included stocking a specific list of products. The Sanidad monitored not just pharmacies' inventories but also the quality of the items stocked and the adequacy of storage conditions (especially for items that required refrigeration). In addition, pharmacies had to follow specific opening hours, since they were a special category of commercial establishment that fulfilled a social function. And as discussed, there were staffing requirements.

Given their investment in medications, equipment, and salaries, pharmacy owners mobilized to prevent the sale of drugs in other kinds of venues. They objected strenuously to the fact that other venders were able to compete with them at a lower cost precisely because they did not have the same obligatory expenses. While in many ways pharmacy owners did not constitute a group—their interests brought them instead into competition with each other—in this particular area they cooperated with each other in lobbying for their sole right to sell various medicinal products, some of which might be available from street vendors or from general stores. For instance, in late 1931, a group of pharmacy owners together petitioned the director of Sanidad "with the objective of prohibiting that various commercial establishments like grocery stores, etc., are converted into drugstores."[43] They specifically pointed out that other businesses could offer patent medicines at a lower cost given that they did not have the additional operating expenses that pharmacies had to incur.[44] In response, the director called a meeting attended by the majority of representatives and owners of Quito's pharmacies to discuss these problems.

The director opened the meeting by reporting that he had ordered the Sanidad comisario to notify shop owners Dolores Cortez and Miguel Proaño that they could not sell medications in their general stores (the issue that had spurred the pharmacy owners' petition). While they were gathered to deal with this item of mutual interest, the Sanidad also had the representatives of the pharmacies agree on a new schedule of turnos. To avoid future problems and resolve past ones, the director had the attendees sign a formal agreement committing to close their businesses at seven o'clock on evenings when they were not de turno as well as on Sundays and civic holidays. This arrangement was then further formalized as an order (*decreto*) of the director of Sanidad, using the provisions of the Código de Policía Sanitaria, so that any infraction would be judged by the comisario of the central zone of Sanidad. Finally, the meeting circled back around to the pharmacy owners' initial concern: "It ended by asking that the Directorate of Sanidad publish in the press a warning that other commercial establishments, under the Ley y Reglamento de Boticas y

Droguerías, are only permitted to sell the following medicinal substances, of domestic and inoffensive use: flaxseed, almond oil, flaxseed oil, orange blossom water, camphor, crystalized alum, star anise, barley sugar [*azucar cande*], sulphur bars, sulphur precipitate, creolin, borage flowers, chamomile flowers, mallow flowers, salsify flowers, elderberry flowers, linden flowers, lavender flowers, mustard, tamarind pulp, sagu palm and tapioca."[45] In this meeting the pharmacy representatives agreed to accept certain restrictions on their own operations provided their direct competitors did the same, while they also ensured that their collective interests were defended against other vendors who were not subject to some of the strict conditions that governed registered pharmacies.

In moments like this, pharmacy owners behaved as a group by together soliciting that the Sanidad defend their collective interests, and the Sanidad in turn treated them as a group by calling them all to a meeting to discuss items of mutual interest. While in some ways owners shared interests, they were largely not a unified group. Indeed, pharmacies of various sizes were clearly positioned differently in terms of their ability to take on certain costs of operating, as botica owner Flor's comments above highlighted. Having successfully worked together to move the sale of drugs out of other venues and into pharmacies, certain key figures then attempted to branch out into new commercial areas within their pharmacies. The entrepreneurial owner of the Botica Pichincha, Eduardo Ledesma de Janón, who established his pharmacy in the late 1930s after buying out the Botica La Protectora, led the way.

The Botica Pichincha opened in a prime location in the heart of the colonial city center, diagonal to the Plaza del Teatro on the northwest corner of Guayaquil and Esmeraldas streets, in a recently constructed art nouveau building that also housed the Hotel Europa. Ledesma's interest in expanding the products on offer at the Botica Pichincha was foreshadowed by his ownership of another venture, the Laboratorio y Perfumería Squirrel, alongside his role as import representative not only for pharmaceutical items but also for a New York company that produced glasswork and hospital implements, a Maryland company that produced chrome items, two companies in Hamburg (one producing paint and varnishes, the other porcelain items), a company in Vienna producing leather goods, and a company in India producing sporting goods (all of which were listed on the crowded margins of his business stationery). The pharmacy inspection commission felt that the Botica Pichincha, to justify its relatively high prices, focused far too much on appearances—with its lotions dispensed in fine porcelain jars and other items in elegant little boxes—and not enough on the quality of its products. However, "the primordial function of a pharmacy is not its commercial aspect, but rather its service to incapacitated humanity, without distinctions between rich and poor," the commission insisted.[46]

Ledesma indeed had a different notion than the inspection commission about the purpose of a pharmacy. He took advantage of special provisions that applied to pharmacies, which again were considered to serve a social function, when he petitioned to ensure his business could stay open for extended hours and on weekends (when the Labor Code normally dictated closure to ensure employees' rights to time off). While as a pharmacy, it did fall under those provisions, a Sanidad official clarified that there was a tacit agreement among the city's pharmacy owners to close when their businesses were not de turno, and on this basis Ledesma's peers had protested against his plans for the Botica Pichincha.[47] Ledesma continued to push the limits of what was permitted. Tensions with the inspectors increased when the Botica Pichincha owner was formally notified of the clause in the Ley de Boticas that stated, "Pharmacies and drugstores are not permitted to sell articles other than medications, chemical products, biologics, essences, and alcohols, instruments and equipment of hygienic, medical or chemical application, or analogous items." Despite this stipulation, the owner of the Botica Pichincha "with an understandable commercial eagerness and no doubt forgetting this clause, offers for sale . . . articles that are entirely foreign to a pharmacy or drugstore," argued the Sanidad.[48] Ledesma explained that in fact in the "droguería" section of his store he only sold pharmaceutical and related products. However, he also had a "bazaar" department which is where he sold "perfumes, sanitary products, razor blades, nail files, etc., etc." He took advantage of the opportunity to also inform the chief of pharmacy inspection that he was delighted to announce that he also planned to introduce an entirely new product the following month: "I will establish a new section, completely independent of the others, where ice cream [*helados hechos a máquina*] will be sold. Since I know you have travelled beyond the narrow borders of our country, I imagine you will view with satisfaction the effort I am making to endow this city with a pharmacy that, going beyond most others in the country, rises to the height of similar businesses in other more cultured centers that under the name of '*Drugstores*' [in English in the original] offer a complete service to society."[49]

The chief inspector referred this situation to his supervisor, and it was the regional director of Sanidad who responded with an order instructing Ledesma not to proceed with his plan. Predictably, Ledesma then contacted the minister of social welfare and labor. He explained that by initiating the sale of pasteurized ice cream, he was aspiring to displace the street sale of ice cream made with unboiled water and contaminated milk, which the Sanidad director himself had identified as a source of typhoid. Ledesma sought just a temporary permit to continue his service until a new Ley de Boticas, which was currently being debated, could be passed. And as Ledesma hoped, the new law was passed the following year and contained explicit permission to sell ice cream. After listing the pharmaceutical items to be sold, Article 9 of the law added "any pharmacy whose locale and hygienic conditions permit, may establish separate sections such as soda and ice cream fountains, as long as the preparation and sale of these items does not interfere with the dispensing of medication."[50]

These ongoing tussles illuminate some of the limits of the Sanidad's institutional power. While they had many successes in managing conflicts among pharmacies where they primarily had to balance similar interests, they struggled to assert their authority over a well-connected and ambitious entrepreneur with a different vision for his enterprise (who also adeptly used Sanidad officials' own language against them). Time would confirm that Ledesma's vision was the future of Ecuadorian pharmacy businesses: after he sold Botica Pichincha to the owners of Botica Quito in 1950, it was one of the foundational pieces of what became Farmacias y Boticas Ecuatorianas Compañía Anónima, or FYBECA, in 1965, now the largest pharmacy chain in the country, carrying a very wide range of products. The former Botica Pichincha locale in the city center continues to be a prized possession for the chain.

A rather different large-scale entrepreneurial initiative relevant to drug preparation was also established during this period. In the context of shortages associated with the onset of the Second World War, a group of Ecuadorians came together in June 1940 to establish Laboratorios Industriales Farmaceúticos Ecuatorianos (L.I.F.E., or Ecuadorian Industrial Pharmaceutical Laboratories). The founding of L.I.F.E. "has as its objective the fabrication of chemical-pharmaceutical products, products of organic chemistry synthesis, vitamins, Galenic preparations, dietic products and products for radiological uses." The locale was adjacent to the Hospital Eugenio Espejo, occupying a complex of ten thousand square meters, furnished with modern equipment from Europe and the US along with some machinery made in Ecuador. The technical staff included ten experienced physicians, chemists, and pharmacists. In addition to laboratory analyses to ensure the purity of all substances used in their preparations, L.I.F.E. also carried out both clinical trials and laboratory tests to verify the therapeutic efficacy of their products. The establishment of L.I.F.E. was clearly framed as a project of import substitution industrialization: "We are sure that within a relatively short period of time, Ecuador will be free of the need to import any pharmaceutical product, and even more, the country will be in a position to export medical products." They also hoped both to reduce imports of prime materials and to explore export possibilities for medicinal plants cultivated in Ecuador, explaining that "by means of the broad possibilities available to us, we have initiated already the study of how we might take advantage of the many items with medicinal properties that Ecuador produces, with the goal that we will be able, for the good of the country itself, to see ourselves freed, for the production of medications, from the importation of prime materials from abroad as much as possible; and also to organize in the country the production and collection of medicinal plants for export, with enormous advantages for the national economy."[51] In the following months, L.I.F.E. was indeed certified to export its pharmaceutical products to Venezuela (November 1942), Guatemala (April 1943), El Salvador (January 1944), and Bolivia (April 1944).

L.I.F.E. did not sell its products directly to the general public, but it did increase the availability of patent medicines produced, for the first time, within the country. This could be beneficial to pharmacy owners in increasing their access and lowering prices, but it also increased the availability of these products for sale in droguerías (where medications were sold but not prepared), which sometimes competed with pharmacies. As with so many of the processes explored here, the establishment of L.I.F.E. had multiple and sometimes contradictory effects, changing the terrain on which pharmacy owners operated and how they competed with other kinds of vendors as well as with each other.

This large-scale project to process and commercialize natural medicinal products may also be related to a new Sanidad order that came a few years later to cancel all permits for ambulant sales of all "chemical-pharmaceutical products or those coming from the Región Oriental [Eastern or Amazon region]. . . . The holders or introducers of medicinal products coming from the Región Oriental can only sell them in the pharmacies or laboratories legally established in the Sanidad central zone."[52] The rationale was, again, that "only in the pharmacies can the effectiveness of a product be proven, not in grocery stores and certainly not among ambulant vendors."[53] Both L.I.F.E. and pharmacies were positioned to benefit from bringing these additional therapeutic resources into their domains.

As it moved into the administrative space of monitoring who could prescribe, who could dispense, and who could sell drugs and medicinal preparations, the Sanidad encountered a rich set of conflicts that required mediation. The Sanidad registered the credentials of physicians; distributed nóminas to pharmacies so they wouldn't accept unlicensed practitioners' prescriptions; used these same provisions to monitor other practitioners (like midwives); investigated and fined unlicensed practitioners; authorized other kinds of medical practice where physicians were absent but then put those people out of business when a licensed practitioner arrived; and simultaneously monitored physicians and defended their professional rights. While pharmacists, in turn, were those assigned rights to dispense medications, here too there were a number of ways that regulations addressed potential conflicts of interest or of commitment that could cause pharmacist shortages. These provided an opening for practitioners with less formal training to receive permission to dispense drugs, permits that could be both issued and revoked by the Sanidad. Because of the Sanidad's role in providing these approvals and monitoring unlicensed practitioners, it also became a central point in the lobbying efforts of pharmacy students and recent graduates to secure positions. Finally, the sale of drugs also required monitoring and mediation since pharmacy owners had special requirements for their pharmacy operations that other commercial enterprises did not: employment of qualified pharmacists, reliable refrigeration, maintenance of a specific inventory of medicinal components and products, and so on. These responsibilities were balanced out by the exclusive rights these establishments had to prepare complex medications and use narcotics in their prescriptions.[54]

What is striking in the documentation is the many different groups whose paths intersected in this dimension of Sanidad activity. In the various activities involved in prescribing, dispensing, and selling drugs, the Sanidad simultaneously monitored practitioners and pharmacies and defended their professional and commercial rights. It was positioned at the center of a Venn diagram of conflicting demands and interests, and it achieved considerable success in making itself essential to their resolution. Where Sanidad officials seemed to be most effective was where they could balance different interests in a way that offered something to all parties, making it easier to cajole (rather than force) the parties into compliance as they could see advantages for themselves in how these matters were resolved. Rather than seeing the political instability of the 1930s as posing obstacles to the smooth functioning of this system, we might more productively see it as a means by which Sanidad officials came to the fore as social processes were activated to make the legal provisions on paper real in people's lives. This reminds us that passing a law, as political geographer Joe Painter pointed out, has little immediate effect on its own.[55] It comes into being—it is realized or made real—through the practices of many social actors combining sufficiently to permit administrative action. Beyond this important conceptual point, for the Sanidad in particular this created a proliferation of contexts where they were called upon to explain policies, gather information, and negotiate among different groups. Sometimes, they even had to clarify the landscape of policy and practice to newly appointed cabinet ministers, who had to rely on Sanidad officials' knowledge and experience perhaps more than would normally be the case, given their short terms in office. Just as there was never a crisis that Sanidad officials did not seem to embrace as an opportunity, they also never missed a chance to mediate a conflict and to make themselves central to how a range of people could pursue their interests and resolve their everyday problems.

Conclusions

From its founding in 1908 through to the mid-1940s, the everyday practices of the Ecuadorian Servicio de Sanidad, or Public Health Service, contributed to generating an idea of the state as able to intervene beneficially in people's lives, while it was also expanding its network of personnel over the national territory to enable coordinated action, thus strengthening the state system. State agencies and governing programs can undoubtedly impose significant constraints on people, but this account foregrounds some dimensions of what state activity can facilitate. Governing processes and projects always work to enable something for someone—equally when opportunities and resources are provided and when regulations are being dismantled. The more that the enabling processes align with certain groups' own aspirations, the more compelling and legitimating they become. As diverse members of Ecuadorian society engaged with public health programs, the projects themselves might be reshaped through the back-and-forth of petition, response, appeal, and so on. Active engagement by a variety of social actors might push the limits of what was intended in establishing those programs, revealing both the uncertain and contingent outcomes of state initiatives and the importance of nonstate actors in making the state real.

The word *encounters* used in this book's title points to the ways that, in the processes discussed here, the paths of diverse social actors intersected at moments that both were snapshots in time and formed part of ongoing relationships and historical processes. Under ideal conditions, an analysis of the moment of encounter would include an understanding of the previous experiences, varied intentions, and aspirations for the future that the various actors brought to their encounter. It could make a difference who the specific person was who tried to advance a project, if he or she had a good reputation with colleagues, strong connections with other institutional actors, or an openness to compromise in order to better meet the needs of the population targeted by a project. Perhaps this became less important over time as institutional structures themselves became more robust. While that ideal analysis is difficult to achieve, nonetheless an appreciation for these multiple dimensions can help deepen our understanding of how people's past experiences, perceptions, and motivations may be orienting their actions as recorded—only ever partially—in the archival record.

This kind of analysis requires, in equal measure, careful archival research and an imaginative leap that allows us to envision ourselves in those encounters, including imagining not knowing the outcome or future trajectory of events. What was it like, for instance, to work on plague eradication while the means of transmission were still being clarified and the most effective interventions in a location were unclear? Foregrounding experience is aided by immersion in uncatalogued archival material in a way that resembles ethnographic fieldwork. Rather than permitting a targeted search for specific documents, the character of the archives lent itself to following the ebb and flow of correspondence and records to develop a feel for the general shape of relations and activities, including the unexpected challenges and emerging divergences and alignments as well as the intended outcomes. An advantage of using correspondence among a wide variety of state agents affiliated with different agencies or differently positioned within a single agency is that one can have no illusion that state actors were working smoothly and harmoniously toward a shared goal.

The processes analyzed here highlight the importance of trust for public health measures. Internalized trust at the level of belief cannot be assessed nor should it be assumed, but the archival sources do offer evidence of the outward manifestations of people's behavior that they hoped, or at least calculated, that public health employees could help them resolve difficulties. When Quito subdirector of Sanidad Dr. Carlos Miño asserted in 1920 that the public health service had "deeply entered the minds of the people and . . . rooted itself in their habits,"[1] it is the latter point that may be most important. It was their habits that could alter the trajectory of disease transmission, but in addition, their behavior in reaching out to the Sanidad service to resolve difficulties is another essential element of practice for understanding the growing capacity of the state to intervene. As Amy Cooper reminds us in her ethnography of healthcare in Chávez's Venezuela,[2] while anthropologists have often leaned toward doing "dark anthropology" emphasizing suffering, there is much to be gained from exploring processes with more positive outcomes (even if only partially so). My research in Ecuador has been shaped since I began to study the region by wondering what constellation of social and political processes kept Ecuador from experiencing the kind of civil conflict that occurred in several other Latin American countries in the 1980s. In this book, I continued to explore the processes contributing to a partially successful hegemonic project that permitted the incorporation of some aspirations of subordinate groups into practices of governing.[3] In the context of public health, the notion of care is helpful for understanding these dynamics as a broader approach beyond treatment for a specific illness. If we extend care to mean something like a willingness to dignify people's concerns or show sufficient empathy to be able to grasp their situation and hence facilitate solving certain everyday dilemmas, then this capacity seems to have contributed to how public health officials' actions helped conjure the state.

There are many ways to think about care in relation to public health, and Lisa Stevenson highlights some of the costs of too much care of the kind that the Canadian state offered to (or imposed on) Inuit people in the northern territory of Nunavut.[4] Her analysis facilitates thinking comparatively, which helps clarify some of the distinctive features of the Ecuadorian context. Stevenson writes of a biopolitics of care that operated at a population level with an aggressively paternalistic project of improving the Inuit population in ways that turned people into statistics and detached them from their networks of relationships. This was expressed through programs to remove tuberculosis patients from their families and their communities for treatment in southern Canada. These patients might never be heard from again. She also writes of the neutrality of care that could itself be perceived as oppressive through erasing personal relationships between state agents and the targets of their programs. As her research participants put it, this might lead people to "take it personally" when state agents set aside relationships built through other programs when they felt they needed to inhabit a more punitive role, which generated a sense of betrayal.

In comparison to what Stevenson describes, Ecuadorian state agents were not able to institute the dense "statification" of social life that was sometimes possible in North America and Europe,[5] and in particular they could not easily penetrate the countryside where most of the Indigenous population continued to reside in the early twentieth century. There was not sufficient critical mass of public health officials (and there were few physicians in general outside Ecuador's three largest cities) to allow them to compete with other influential people already occupying that terrain. The latter is an important point, as colonial and postcolonial economic projects in Ecuador were built on the intensive use of Indigenous labor in agricultural and textile production, which led to dense configurations of power relations in rural areas. In particular, within large agricultural estates there could be direct intrusion by *hacienda* owners and administrators in intimate life, for instance when a peasant tenant wished to marry (which had direct implications for the possibilities to extract labor and the size of peasant usufruct plots, both relevant for the operations of the hacienda). More recently, anthropologist Christopher Krupa observes that in the early twenty-first century some modernizing Ecuadorian landowners producing cut flowers for the international market took on a "state by proxy" role when they stepped in to provide services that the government was still not capable of sustaining.[6] In doing so, they fostered new forms of dependency among rural workers, which are of a different character than earlier ties of paternalism and dependence on rural estates, but equally occupied spaces that were thereby lost to state agents. The Ecuadorian countryside was and continues to be a terrain in dispute when it comes to forms of governing.

In the Guaytacama plague outbreak discussed in chapter 1, large landowners supported the Sanidad campaign and vowed to ensure the cooperation of the Indigenous peasants on their estates. This could easily have become another arena where their relations with state agents amplified landowners' power. However, Sanidad officials seized on the opportunity to demonstrate that they were not susceptible to landowner pressures and that they had an uncompromising attitude toward local power holders. This is what allowed them to seem to stand over and apart from society and, in doing so, to maintain sufficient distance from local elites to comprehend and respond to the concerns of Indigenous peasants (who were both laborers recruited for the anti-plague campaign and targets of vaccination efforts). While their success was due partly to the specific skills and attitudes of the Sanidad officials involved, there were also structural features of the situation that lent themselves to these outcomes. The creation of a state system made up of national officials who extended their reach across the national territory with a mandate to protect the health of the national population over private or individual interests might have special meaning where the private interests to be subordinated included those of influential local elites. This built on public health messaging in other areas that emphasized the need to subordinate individual rights to the larger social good, by means of which Sanidad officials were constructing notions of the collective interest—society—as well as of the state.

There is much room for additional research on whether other disease elimination campaigns that took Sanidad physicians into rural areas had similar features, and under what conditions they produced the same social effects. David Carey Jr.'s new research comparing racial dynamics in Guatemalan and Ecuadorian disease elimination campaigns promises new insights by bringing a comparative perspective to these issues.[7] In rural areas, it may be that other Ecuadorian state agents were more likely to play the role of standing over society and intervening in it. In the Juliana period and into the 1930s, for instance, the inspectors who investigated labor complaints on rural estates may have had similar opportunities to mediate local relations as the Sanidad did in the country's more urban spaces.[8]

While Sanidad leaders largely seemed to avoid racializing the health issues they were confronting in the first two decades of the agency's operations—and they framed their general communications in terms of broad parameters of healthy behavior—nonetheless their interventions took place in racialized contexts. This was clear in both encounters examined in chapter 1 on Ecuadorian plague experiences. Recruitment of day laborers for municipal public works—the mechanism that was used during and after the 1913 plague outbreaks to bring laborers to the Alausí cantonal seat to carry out disinfection and other measures put in place by the Sanidad—preferentially sought out Indigenous laborers based on long-standing practices. Similarly, the hacienda system in Guaytacama undoubtedly had a racialized labor regime, although public health campaigns in the area were not framed in this way. The explicitly anti-Indigenous language in a published document by a public health official in 1943 strikes one as unusual in that context (see chapter 1).[9] The intensity of monitoring at the time was also unprecedented and was only possible due to international funding: in that year, 189,048 rural domestic inspections took place among the Indigenous population in Chimborazo province. Perhaps access to more technical fixes to address plague—cyanide gas and flamethrowers—made establishing empathetic relations with Indigenous peasants seem less important to the success of eradication campaigns.[10] Importantly, this pathologization and surveillance of the Indigenous population occurred in a changed political environment, with the emergence of new alliances between rural and urban workers and the 1944 foundation of the first Indigenous federation, the Federación Ecuatoriana de Indios (FEI). Despite the contemptuous words of the anti-plague section chief in chapter 1, the threat posed by Indigenous people might not have been primarily due to their distance from Ecuadorian national society after all.

The question of how states rule focuses our attention on how rule is achieved. Importantly, the history of public health in Ecuador highlights ways that protagonism is not only on the side of state actors. Those figures sometimes seemed to be consciously trying to forge a state system and a new state idea, both of which contributed to setting the terms of engagement with nonstate actors from a variety of social groups. But attention should also be paid to how actions by diverse groups within the recipient or target population can call the state into being in new contexts. As Krupa argues, it is "the ever-dynamic relays of claim and recognition that insinuate state power into the material relations of everyday life."[11] In the account presented here, in many situations it required action by other social actors to set in motion state agents' capacity to intervene. This was made possible by the establishment of specific state programs, positions, or channels of communication through which claims could be pressed or assistance sought: in other words, the extension of the state system was crucial for the possibility of deepening the state idea. For instance, new regulations about domestic waste disposal in Quito might set off a chain of complaints about neighbors, inspections, fines, appeals of the penalties to higher authorities, further responses, and so on. Each step provided an opportunity not only for residents to seek the assistance of state agents but also for Sanidad officials to emphasize their key role in managing these conflicts and, at the same time, extend the framing of problems from the impact of one person's decisions on adjacent properties to the need to protect the health of an entire neighborhood. When it came to installation of toilets, domestic inspections by the service led to citations for violations, followed by appeals of those fines because residents couldn't follow the regulations without access to fixtures or services, answered by successful negotiations by the Sanidad with the municipality, which generated the conditions for complying with regulations. Complaints from tenants about their landlords brought public health officials into cross-class relations in ways that further legitimated their authority. With the marked paternalism characterizing Ecuadorian cross-class social relations, Sanidad officials successfully inserted themselves as good and perhaps more neutral patrons, disrupting and interfering with direct relations of dependency.

Much of the material in this book reflected an urban social dynamic and addressed a diverse population of urban dwellers. This also shows some of the limits of these processes. If a medium-sized city like Ambato (with about fifteen thousand inhabitants) had a more constrained social environment in which the Sanidad delegate struggled to stand apart from local social relations, one can imagine how much more difficult this would be in smaller towns in the Andes. More deeply embedded local officials could not easily achieve sufficient distance from social dynamics to conjure the state, unlike what seemed possible in a city like Quito or when national officials arrived from afar to visit provincial areas. Distance from the local might be a precondition to generate a state effect of standing over and apart from society, suggesting the importance of spatial dynamics in these processes.

This historical ethnography of the Ecuadorian public health agency also draws attention to other important questions in understanding how states rule. How do state actors combine their efforts effectively with each other to enable any kind of action? How do they communicate; issue orders; and generate, circulate and retain records? How do they manage relations with other state or quasi-state agencies at different scales or with adjacent mandates? These all turned out to be difficult tasks in highland Ecuador, and likely elsewhere too. Recent experience with the COVID-19 pandemic further highlights the importance of how different agencies share information and combine their efforts and the many obstacles to effective action. The difficulty of persuading the public in real time of the nature of a health threat and the best ways to combat it, as knowledge of both of those dimensions continues to morph, should not be underestimated. How things get done—a key question for political anthropology—merits more attention in both the present and the past.

This material also raises some questions about what political instability might concretely mean for state formation.[12] Does it just point to a failed or weak state? For lobbying purposes, political instability that led to frequent changes in cabinet ministers could open up new opportunities to press for advantage, as we saw in chapter 5. And this in turn could offer additional occasions requiring mediation of competing interests or the deeper institutional memory that the Sanidad had. In Ecuador, while there was rapid turnover in high offices (including in the executive branch and at the ministry level) there was considerably more stability of personnel within the Sanidad service. This is significant because ongoing relationships within and between agencies, as well as with the public, made a difference in the functioning of the office. But in addition, instability at the highest levels of government may have enhanced the perception that effective action could more likely be expected at the agency level than from the national government. And it also made political appointees more dependent on seasoned agency leaders; with such rapid turnover, they themselves couldn't always acquire enough experience in their roles to carry out their duties effectively. This might have deepened a perception of a stable and more reliable state versus unstable and more fleeting government regimes.

This early account of how Ecuadorian public health conjured the state reminds us that processes of developing both a more robust state system and a perception of a functional and helpful state are not unilineal. Advances in strengthening the institutional structure in the 1920s could be partially undermined in the 1930s by economic crisis, even if the associated political instability had unpredictable and mixed effects.

And in the 1940s, the more inclusive language from the 1920s of some state agents seemed on the wane as the increasing political involvement of Indigenous social actors might generate backlash. The COVID-19 pandemic is a painful reminder that coordination is difficult, trust is fragile, and equity is a continuing and urgent challenge both within and between countries. Stopping this narrative at a different historical moment might suggest that public health was triumphant, when in fact Ecuador's COVID-19 pandemic response shows how many weaknesses there continue to be. Importantly, one could say the same about most countries' responses to COVID-19, including their capacity to coordinate within and between agencies and levels of government and their ability to comprehend the diverse effects on different social groups of each element of their programs. Recent experience also highlights how crucial it is to understand the political and social processes embedded in and around public health campaigns alongside evolving scientific knowledge of disease, whether in the past, present, or future.

Notes

Introduction

1. Eskey, "Chief Etiological Factors," 2083.

2. Clark, "Indians, the State and Law."

3. Clark, *Redemptive Work*, chap. 7. When I was doing doctoral archival research in Alausí in the early 1990s, Nisag community members could still make the authorities scramble when they arrived en masse in government offices to demand their rights.

4. This perspective is influenced by Max Gluckman's early work in political anthropology. In his classic article nicknamed "The Bridge," Gluckman undertakes an "event analysis" of an encounter among a variety of Zululander groups, together comprising the region's "Black-White community," who were all motivated to attend a bridge inauguration ceremony for different reasons. He then unpacks the underlying processes that influenced their interactions, including one that doesn't appear on the surface of the event description—the power of the colonial state. Gluckman, "Analysis."

5. While this seems like a simple idea, it is rarely fully realized. Among cultural history studies of Ecuador that attempt an approach of this kind, Ernesto Capello's *City at the Center* stands out for its unusually rich contextualization of the social landscape.

6. Andrés Guerrero brings attention to some of these issues in his influential study "Una imagen ventrílocua," where he highlights how Indigenous peasants parroted back to the liberal state its discourse about them.

7. Abrams, "Notes on the Difficulty," 79, 82 (emphasis added). This article was written in 1977 and published a decade later in the first issue of the journal inspired by his work.

8. Corrigan and Sayer, *Great Arch*.

9. Relevant to this question, Jean-Paul Deler's attention to the increase in administrative units in Ecuador (provinces, cantons, and civil parishes), and therefore also the density of state officials, is essential reading (*Ecuador*, 187–92).

10. Abrams, "Notes on the Difficulty," 76, 82.

11. Joseph and Nugent, *Everyday Forms.*

12. Mallon, *Peasant and Nation*; and Grandin, *Blood of Guatemala.*

13. Coronel, "Revolution in Stages"; and Coronel, *La última guerra.*

14. Ospina Peralta, *La aleación inestable.*

15. Krupa and Nugent, *State Theory.*

16. Gramsci, "Notes on Italian History"; Clark, *Redemptive Work*; and Clark, "Language of Contention."

17. Drinot, *Allure of Labor.*

18. Smith, *Institutional Ethnography.*

19. Painter, "Prosaic Geographies."

20. Painter, "Prosaic Geographies," 761. Also helpful on these points is John Clarke's identification of the different kinds of labor brought together in the work of governing ("Work of Governing").

21. Painter, "Prosaic Geographies," 768.

22. Painter, "Prosaic Geographies," 757. Similarly, in an otherwise suggestive article, Michel-Rolph Trouillot also highlights Abrams's state idea—in his case without mentioning the state system—and argues that "Abrams's state-idea is not immediately conducive to ethnography" ("Anthropology of the State," 127). This seems a missed opportunity for both authors.

23. Mitchell, "Limits of the State," 86.

24. Painter, "Prosaic Geographies," 758.

25. Painter, "Prosaic Geographies," 771.

26. Farmer, *Fevers, Feuds, and Diamonds.*

27. Farmer, *Fevers, Feuds, and Diamonds*, 33.

28. Compatible with this general approach, Amy Cooper presents a recent case in her study of the pleasure that Venezuelans take in the health activities promoted and extended by Chávez's Bolivarian revolution, especially through the Barrio Adentro program (*State of Health*).

29. This became clear, for instance, when they felt some of their subordinate employees (public health midwives) were acting in ways they disparaged, as midwives struggled to implement policies on the ground (Clark, *Gender, State, and Medicine*, chap. 4; and Clark, "New Arenas").

30. Wolf, *Geografía y geología*, 45–46. All translations from Spanish to English are my own.

31. Dawson, *South American Republics*, 341.

32. The word "creole" indicates European ancestry but birth in the Americas.

33. These were overwhelmingly located in the highlands. Indeed, at the beginning of the twentieth century just 53 of a total 458 churches in Ecuador were in the coastal region, and only 6 of 47 convents (Mena Villamar, *Ecuador a comienzos*, 26).

34. Ronn Pineo's early work on health problems and health care in Guayaquil continues to be useful ("Misery and Death").

35. See Cueto, *Value of Health*, chap. 3.

36. Cumming, "Commercial and Sanitary Relations," 2130. See also "Panama: Plague Conditions." For a description of the hardship to travelers caused by the lack of quarantine facilities along the west coast, see de León and Harman, "Lack of Quarantine Stations."

37. "Ecuador: Health and Sanitary Condition," 861–62.

38. The destroyed buildings included the hospital; the Junta de Beneficencia moved quickly to build a new Hospital General, inaugurated two years later (Pineo, "Misery and Death," 625).

39. "Ecuador: Health and Sanitary Condition," 864.

40. While normally urban yellow fever is not considered gender-selective, in Guayaquil nearly all of the victims were male (Pineo, *Social and Economic Reform*, 103), perhaps because of the influx of nonimmune laborers from elsewhere. In 1897, for instance, the reconstruction of the city following the previous year's fire employed 2,500 day laborers (Ibarra, *Indios y cholos*, 9–10).

41. Cornejo Gómez, "Informe del Delegado," 346, 349.

42. A fourth disease covered by international sanitary agreements, cholera, did not affect Ecuador during the era covered in this book.

43. Cornejo Gómez, "Informe del Delegado," 348.

44. A partial solution came a few years later, when a hospital was established in Milagro, inland from Guayaquil, to treat local patients afflicted with yellow fever and other diseases. By the middle of 1915, the building had been completed but there were not yet any operating funds available to open it. The director general estimated that about six hundred patients annually from this zone were being treated in Guayaquil facilities (Becerra, "Informe del Director de Sanidad," 505). The Milagro hospital was inaugurated in March 1917.

45. The loss of the Guayaquil Sanidad's office and archive in a fire in October 1917 also prevents an analysis of the everyday practices of that office for the first decade of its functioning. The record of Guayaquil officials' correspondence with Quito officials is preserved in the Archivo del Servicio de Sanidad in Quito, but this is only a small portion of what their archive would have held.

46. Capello, *City at the Center*, 12.

47. Williams, "Assembling the 'Empire of Morality.'" Erin O'Connor brings attention to the gendered dimensions of the Garcian project in her book *Gender, Indian, Nation*, chap. 3.

48. The liberal emphasis on movement of people and goods, developed in a range of government projects, is analyzed in detail in Clark, *Redemptive Work*, chap. 3.

49. Parks and Nuermberger, "Sanitation of Guayaquil."

50. Rodríguez, *Search for Public Policy*, continues to be a useful source for

this time period. See also Durán, *Irrupción del sector*; and Paz y Miño Cepeda, *Revolución Juliana.*

51. Coronel, "Revolution in Stages," 851.

52. Coronel, "Revolution in Stages."

53. Ospina Peralta, *La aleación inestable*, pt. 2.

54. Maiguashca, "Los sectores subalternos"; Marchán Romero, "La crisis"; and Maiguashca and North, "Orígenes y significado."

55. Pineo, *Social and Economic Reform*, 3.

56. For more information, see Loewenfeld, "Guayaquil and Quito Railway"; and Clark, *Redemptive Work*, chap. 7.

57. See Clark, *Redemptive Work*, chap. 4.

58. Loewenfeld, "Guayaquil and Quito Railway," 89.

59. Cited in Clark, *Redemptive Work*, 196.

60. Parks and Nuermberger, "Sanitation of Guayaquil," 204–5.

61. See, for instance, Palmer, *Launching Global Health.*

62. These events are described in Parks and Nuermberger, "Sanitation of Guayaquil," 215–19, although the authors' markedly disparaging tone toward Ecuadorians is distracting. Readers of this article would come away believing erroneously that US actors were the main protagonists in the history of Ecuadorian public health.

63. Benedict Anderson highlights similar dynamics in his discussion of the formation of administrative territories (*Imagined Communities*).

64. Ferguson and Gupta, "Spatializing States."

65. Slack, *Plague*, 74.

66. In his comparative analysis of Indigenous healing traditions and scientific medicine in Guatemala and Ecuador, *Health in the Highlands*, David Carey Jr. presents a number of other disease eradication projects undertaken in Ecuador, complementing the discussion of plague presented here with extended analyses of campaigns against other diseases such as malaria.

Chapter 1: Encountering Plague, Plague Encounters

Epigraph: Lloyd, "Plague," 729. In 1908, Lloyd was a US consular official in Guayaquil and led the laboratory identification of the first plague outbreak in Ecuador.

1. The first plague pandemic occurred in the Mediterranean and Europe from around 541 AD to 750 AD (beginning with the "plague of Justinian"). Both the geographical reach and the timeline for the second—the "Black Death"—has been extended by Monica H. Green's ongoing research, combining insights from paleogenetics (or, the "biological archive") with documentary evidence ("Four Black Deaths"). Research is ongoing into all three plague pan-

demics. In addition to Green's work, see also Mordechai and Eisenberg, "Rejecting Catastrophe"; and Slack, "Perceptions of Plague." I have learned a great deal from Christos Lynteris and his colleagues on the research projects "Visual Representations of the Third Plague Pandemic" (2013–2018) and "The Global War against the Rat and the Epistemic Emergence of Zoonosis" (2019–2024), which have significantly expanded the questions being explored about the third pandemic and bring together anthropological and historical perspectives very effectively. In addition to the special journal issue and edited volume cited in note 7 (among many other such contributions), Lynteris and Poleykett's introduction to another journal special issue, "Anthropology of Epidemic Control," provides a good example of the kind of work this group is doing.

2. Echenberg, *Plague Ports*, 15.

3. Moll and O'Leary, "Plague . . . (Part 1)." Because Echenberg's *Plague Ports* narrative ends in 1901, it includes neither the Peruvian nor the Ecuadorian plague histories but does cover the Rio de Janeiro and Buenos Aires outbreaks. For a discussion of plague in Peru, see Cueto, *Return of Epidemics*, chap. 1.

4. Dyl, "War on Rats."

5. "World Prevalence," 196.

6. For leading causes of death in Guayaquil, see Pineo, "Misery and Death."

7. In recent years significant contributions have been made to the anthropological literature on zoonoses. See for instance Keck and Lynteris, "Zoonosis"; and the other contributions to this journal special issue. Many of the essays in Kelly, Keck, and Lynteris's collection *Anthropology of Epidemics* also advance our understanding of zoonoses in important ways, such as Sodikoff's chapter, "Multispecies Infrastructure of Zoonosis."

8. That plague is primarily a rodent rather than a human disease helps to explain why plague is so deadly to humans. Where humans are the primary victims of a disease, a process of taming epidemic diseases by rendering them endemic occurs as an immunological compromise is reached in which (1) the most susceptible individuals die; (2) the most virulent strains of the disease die out because they kill their hosts; and (3) where most hosts survive and can pass on the disease to other hosts, the long process of building up immunities occurs. This has occurred with previously mortal human diseases like measles and chickenpox, which have been transformed into primarily childhood diseases tending to affect children in a milder form than adults and providing them with lifetime immunity. Because humans are not the primary victims of plague, and indeed it affects humans only incidentally, an immunological compromise has not been reached between humans and plague; rather, such a natural process of taming a disease occurs between plague and rats. Where rats do develop partial immunity, then they do not die of plague, and therefore their fleas do not jump off to seek new hosts.

9. Lloyd, "Plague," 731. At the time of his 1925 comments, Lloyd (by then

the assistant surgeon general of the US Public Health Service) considered serum the only available treatment for plague, offering as evidence that during the 1916 outbreak in Alausí, Ecuador, there were eight deaths among the sixty-eight plague patients hospitalized and treated, while all ninety-eight known cases that were not treated died. This paper was initially presented to public health physicians at the 1925 meeting of the American Medical Association, where Lloyd's reflections on Ecuadorian plague experiences, including in the Andean town of Alausí, became part of a larger scientific discussion of the trajectory of plague.

10. "El control," 331–32.

11. Murdock, "Pneumonic Plague." Villagómez had recently left his position as provincial Sanidad delegate to take up the better-paid position of physician for the Caja del Seguro service.

12. Martínez Vinueza, "Peste eruptiva."

13. See Cunningham, "Transforming Plague."

14. "Second General International Sanitary Convention."

15. Echenberg, *Plague Ports*, 58, 62.

16. Pollitzer, *Plague*, 7.

17. World Health Organization, "Health Topics: Plague."

18. The chronology of plague infection given in the following paragraphs is drawn from Miño, *La peste bubónica*.

19. Subdirector of Sanidad for Pichincha to director general of Sanidad, Quito, December 12, 1914, LC-1914, ASS/MNM.

20. Palmer, *Launching Global Health*, emphasizes the importance of the demonstration effect in hookworm campaigns. See also Palmer, *From Popular Medicine*, chap. 7; and Birn, "Revolution."

21. "La pandemia actual," 33.

22. "Ecuador: Reports from Guayaquil."

23. "Ecuador: Report from Quito."

24. See Cueto, *Value of Health*, for a discussion of the role of maritime public health in early Pan-Americanism.

25. Pineo, *Social and Economic Reform*, 124.

26. This was one of many cost-saving shortcuts that made the US-built railway controversial in Ecuador (Clark, *Redemptive Work*, chap. 7).

27. "Parte de los trabajos efectuados por el servicio de fumigación y inspección de carga y equipajes, desde el 10 de junio hasta el 31 de julio de 1916," Ambato, July 31, 1916, LCR-1916, ASS/MNM.

28. By the early 1930s, the Sanidad was in a position to prepare its own *linfa antipestosa*, overseen by Dr. Enrique Sayago Samaniego, laboratory chief in the Guayaquil office, who for instance between April 1930 and April 1931 prepared 11,140 doses distributed primarily to the central and southern zones (where plague was still active at that point). "Informe que el Director de Sanidad

Pública de la Zona del Litoral presenta al Sr. Ministro del Ramo, por medio del Sr. Director General de Sanidad," Guayaquil, May 1931, filed in LCR-Servicio Interno e Informes-1932, ASS/MNM.

29. Director general of Sanidad to the subdirector of Sanidad for Pichincha, Guayaquil, October 21, 1917, LCR-1917, ASS/MNM.

30. A preliminary analysis of Alausí's plague experience is presented in Clark, *Redemptive Work*, chap. 6.

31. In 1909, the population of the town of Alausí and its outskirts (that is, the Alausí parish, within the larger Alausí canton) had been estimated at four thousand. Compañía Guía del Ecuador, *El Ecuador*, 444–45.

32. Clark, "Indians, the State and Law."

33. Director general of Sanidad to the subdirector of Sanidad for Pichincha, Guayaquil, March 19, 1916, LCR-1916, ASS/MNM.

34. Note that in 1909 in the central highland provinces of Chimborazo, Tungurahua, and León, there had only been thirteen physicians practicing in Riobamba (with one in Alausí), four in Ambato, and four in Latacunga. In other words, not only were there few doctors in the provincial capitals, but there was only one licensed physician who was practicing outside a capital in this region. See Compañía Guía del Ecuador, *El Ecuador*, 449, 1109, 1313. While the municipal government in each provincial capital hired a physician to oversee smallpox vaccination, monitor sanitary conditions, and provide some basic medical attention to those with few resources, the services offered were quite limited.

35. Peñaherrera, *Informe . . . 1913*, xiv.

36. President of the municipal council to director of hygiene, Quito, April 26, 1913, LC-Oficina de Higiene Municipal-1913, ASS/MNM.

37. Peñaherrera, *Informe . . . 1914*, xlix.

38. One heated exchange with the railway company manager included descriptions of how, after a piano shipped from Ambato for Miño's personal use had been warehoused for a week in Chimbacalle, rats jumped out of the packing material (Max Meitzner to subdirector of Sanidad, Quito, January 25, 1918, LCR-1918-I, ASS/MNM; subdirector of Sanidad to Max Meitzner, Quito, January 27, 1918, LCE-1918, ASS/MNM).

39. "Informe Anual que el Subdirector de Sanidad de las Provincias de Pichincha, Imbabura y Carchi eleva al Ministerio del Ramo y a la Dirección de Sanidad de Guayaquil, 1919–1920," 6, LCE-1920, ASS/MNM.

40. Printed broadsheet "De Sanidad," Quito, June 5, 1916, LCE-1916, ASS/MNM.

41. Dr. Aurelio Vaca Rosas to the subdirector of Sanidad for Pichincha, Quito, October 22, 1917, LCR-1917, ASS/MNM.

42. Director general of Sanidad to the subdirector of Sanidad for Pichincha, Guayaquil, January 19, 1915, LCR-1915, ASS/MNM.

43. Director general of Sanidad to the subdirector of Sanidad for Pichincha, Guayaquil, November 25, 1915, LCR-1915, ASS/MNM.

44. Train passengers stopped overnight in Riobamba, but the cargo trains themselves did not enter the city, which was connected by a branch line rather than set on the main railway line.

45. "Memorandum de las medidas preventivas que deben adoptarse contra la peste bubónica," subdirector of Sanidad to the minister of the interior and Sanidad, Quito, November 23, 1916, LCE-1916, ASS/MNM.

46. Subdirector of Sanidad for Pichincha to director general of Sanidad, Quito, January 16, 1915, LCE-1915, ASS/MNM.

47. Director general of Sanidad to the subdirector of Sanidad for Pichincha, Guayaquil, December 30, 1920, LCR-1920, ASS/MNM.

48. Director general of Sanidad to the subdirector of Sanidad for Pichincha, Guayaquil, April 17, 1921, LCR-1921, ASS/MNM; director general of Sanidad to the subdirector of Sanidad for Pichincha, Guayaquil, May 13, 1921, LCR-1921, ASS/MNM.

49. Newspaper clipping dated February 8, 1923, enclosed in director general of Sanidad to the subdirector of Sanidad for Pichincha, Guayaquil, February 14, 1923, LCR-1923, ASS/MNM.

50. Director general of Sanidad to minister of public education and Sanidad, Guayaquil, October 27, 1923, LCR-1923, ASS/MNM.

51. Cumming et al, "Pan American Conference," 2592. It was only five years later in 1931 that researchers in India, the country hardest hit by the third plague pandemic, carried out similar work there (Echenberg, *Plague Ports*, 70).

52. Director general of Sanidad to Dr. Samuel B. Grubbs of the Pan American Sanitary Bureau, Quito, February 2, 1927, LCE-1927, ASS/MNM.

53. Cueto, "Andean Biology." Indeed later, in 1941, Ecuador's plague campaigns were lauded: "The lessons learned from the Ecuadorian campaigns have been of value to workers elsewhere. It may have been because of this apparently prevalent spirit of scientific curiosity that Ecuador is one of the countries which has shown the least tendency to ever debate the question as to whether plague has appeared in a given locality—demonstrating an attitude of frankness and fair dealing which deserves full recognition" (Moll and O'Leary, "Plague . . . [Part 12]," 374).

54. Sanidad delegate for Chimborazo to the director general of Sanidad, Riobamba, July 13, 1926, LCR-Delegaciones Provinciales-1926/27, ASS/MNM.

55. The following draws on a shorter account of this outbreak presented in Clark, "New Arenas."

56. The history of agricultural modernization in this region is analyzed in Arcos and Marchán, "Apuntes."

57. For more information about the Sociedad Nacional de Agricultura, see Arcos, "El espíritu del progreso."

58. Various documents from May–July 1926, LC-La Bubónica en Ambato y Guaytacama-1926/27, ASS/MNM.

59. See Clark, *Gender, State, and Medicine*, chap. 3.

60. Pedro Zambrano to the director general of Sanidad, Guaytacama, May 31, 1926, LC-La Bubónica en Ambato y Guaytacama-1926/27, ASS/MNM.

61. Pedro Zambrano to the director general of Sanidad, Guaytacama, June 4, 1926, LC-La Bubónica en Ambato y Guaytacama-1926/27, ASS/MNM.

62. Pedro Zambrano to the director general of Sanidad, Guaytacama, July 6, 1926, LC-La Bubónica en Ambato y Guaytacama-1926/27, ASS/MNM.

63. Sanidad delegate for León to the director general of Sanidad, Latacunga, July 6, 1926, LC-La Bubónica en Ambato y Guaytacama-1926/27, ASS/MNM.

64. Director general of Sanidad to municipal police, Quito, July 19, 1926, LCE-1926, ASS/MNM.

65. Director general of Sanidad to President Ayora, Quito, June 15, 1926, LCE-1926, ASS/MNM.

66. Annual report of Sanidad delegate for Tungurahua from 1 April to 31 December 1926, Ambato, December 31, 1926, LCR-Delegaciones Provinciales-1926/27, ASS/MNM.

67. The Sanidad continued to conduct domestic inspections in 1931 to verify whether Indigenous peasants in Guaytacama were still using these sleeping platforms (Sanidad delegate for León to director general of Sanidad, Latacunga, May 12, 1931, LCR-Direcciones y Delegaciones Provinciales-1931, ASS/MNM).

68. See various documents and petitions from April, May, June, October, and November 1927 in LC-La Bubónica en Ambato y Guaytacama-1926/27, ASS/MNM.

69. See for instance "Campañas Antipestosas en el Ecuador y el Perú" in "Informe Anual del Director de la Oficina Sanitaria Panamericana para el año económico que termina el 30 de junio de 1931," LCR-Oficina Sanitaria Panamericana-1931, ASS/MNM.

70. Long, "Choice of Rat Poison."

71. "Guayaquil, puerto limpio."

72. Telegram from provincial delegate for Loja transcribed in minister of social welfare to director general of Sanidad, Quito, June 4, 1929, LCR-Poder Legislativo/Presidencia de la República/Ministerios/Poder Judicial-1929, ASS/MNM.

73. "Informe Anual presentado por el Delegado de Sanidad de Loja," Loja, December 31, 1930, LC-Informes Anuales de las Delegaciones-1928/30, ASS/MNM.

74. Benjamín Wandemberg to director general of Sanidad, Quito, November 15, 1929, LC-Epidemiología/Servicio Interno-1929, ASS/MNM.

75. Perhaps unsurprisingly, a study of Ecuadorian archives provides a very different picture from that appearing in the US press: the *New York Times*, for instance, in celebrating the eradication of plague in Guayaquil, asserted erroneously that "very little was accomplished until Drs. J. D. Long and C. R. Eskey of the United States Public Health Service started their war on rats last year" ("Guayaquil Has Lost Place").

76. John Long, "Memorandum sobre la peste bubónica en el Ecuador," Quito, December 24, 1929, LC-Epidemiología/Servicio Interno-1929, ASS/MNM.

77. "Guayaquil inscrito," 439.

78. For more information on black and brown rat populations in Guayaquil, see the helpful discussion by Gade, *Nature and Culture*, chap. 8, on which this paragraph draws.

79. Long, "La campaña antipestosa," 927.

80. Sáenz Vera, "Brote de peste," 42.

81. On the nursing school, see Clark, *Gender, State, and Medicine*, chap. 5.

82. Sáenz Vera, "Campaña antipestosa intensiva."

83. Sáenz Vera, "Campaña antipestosa intensiva," 880.

84. See Archetti, *El mundo social.*

85. Sáenz Vera, "Campaña antipestosa intensiva," 881.

86. See Arcos and Marchán, "Apuntes para una discusión."

87. On the Sociedad Nacional de Agricultura and the Law of Agricultural Development, see Clark, *Redemptive Work*, chap. 5.

88. Farmer, *AIDS and Accusation.*

89. See for instance, Suárez, *Contribución al estudio.* For analyses of his research, see Clark, "Race, 'Culture' and Mestizaje"; Prieto, *Liberalismo y temor*; and Kingman Garcés, *La ciudad*, chap. 7.

90. In his new book comparing race and medicine in Guatemala and Ecuador (*Health in the Highlands*), David Carey Jr. argues that disease eradication programs targeting Indigenous people in Guatemala were marked by a darker history of racialization than in Ecuador, consistent with my argument.

91. See the discussion by Cueto and Palmer of DDT use in malaria campaigns in *Medicine and Public Health*, 144–47, 261–62. A reliance on technical fixes over improvements to living conditions is highlighted in their concept of the "culture of survival" characterizing official responses to epidemics in Latin America.

92. In the case he examines of research into the rat's role in plague in India in the early twentieth century, Evans argues that "the industrial work enacted upon rat bodies rendered them into mechanical links: connections with no mo-

rality, such that the whole moral burden of the disease could be shifted to the human realm" ("Blaming the Rat?" 38).

93. Becker, *Indians and Leftists*; Coronel, "Revolution in Stages"; and Clark, "Racial Ideologies."

94. Clarke, "Work of Governing," 212.

Chapter 2: Forging Public Health as State Idea and State System

Epigraph: Ayora, *Informe*, xlvii.

1. Abrams, "Notes on the Difficulty," 79–82.

2. Abbott, *System of Professions*.

3. Official communications directed to a ministry identified the subsection within the ministry that the memo should be channeled to, for instance addressed to "Ministro de lo Interior y Sanidad" when it involved public health.

4. De Lapierre, *Informe*, 9.

5. A broad discussion of key elements of liberal government discourse about progress is presented in Clark, *Redemptive Work*, chap. 3.

6. Valverde, *Informe*, 8.

7. Kingman Garcés (*La ciudad*, 286) mentions briefly in a footnote that a Consejo Superior de Sanidad e Higiene was established in Quito in 1903.

8. Córdova, *Informe*, 10.

9. Puga, *Informe*, xvii.

10. The 1904 law appears to have had the joint goals of preventing religious orders from using their surplus funds to finance counterrevolutionary movements and ensuring the productive use of rural properties to contribute to national progress. It followed on much rhetoric about the accumulation of church wealth by means of exactions from the population, as suggested in this chapter. Initially the liberal government had simply proposed that, given the wealth produced by the agricultural estates owned by religious orders, clergy should not collect fees from the population for various services such as baptism (De Lapierre, *Informe*, 19–23). By 1908, this had escalated to the seizure and nationalization of the estates of foreign religious orders.

11. See for instance Milton, *Many Meanings of Poverty*.

12. As I have explored elsewhere, the Hermanas de la Caridad (Sisters of Charity) religious order continued to administer social welfare institutions under the auspices of the state—indeed, the Hermanas were distinct from all other Catholic orders in that they had come to the country under contract with the government in the 1860s specifically to administer state healthcare institutions (Clark, *Gender, State, and Medicine*, chap. 5).

13. The history of the JBG is explored in depth in Torre, *La Junta*.

14. Rodas Chaves, *Pensamiento médico*, 43.

15. By 1927, the JBG's income solely from rental of this land was greater than the income available to the municipality itself for all of its programs; three years later, part of this property was sold to the government for construction of the Guayaquil airport. See Rojas M. and Villavicencio, *El proceso urbano*, 30–31, 74, 215.

16. Funds generated by the lottery were dedicated to the activities of the JBG by congressional decree; the first lottery draw occurred in November 1894. While there was a decree in 1910 to allow a local lottery in Quito to support Beneficencia activities there, Rodas Chaves argues that opposition from Guayaquil prevented the establishment of a separate lottery in Quito (*Pensamiento médico*, 57).

17. The text of the law is reproduced in Compañía Guía del Ecuador, *El Ecuador*, 225–26.

18. Moncayo, *Informe . . . 1899*, 13. See also Moncayo, *Informe . . . 1898*, 19–20.

19. Importantly, a system of leasing rural estates to large agriculturalists was established, which provided both predictable streams of income to the Juntas de Beneficencia and the opportunity for the leaseholders to accumulate wealth when the negotiated lease payments fell below actual income from the estates.

20. Alfaro, "Message."

21. Reyes V., *Informe*, xvi–xix.

22. Díaz, *Informe*, xxii–xxiv.

23. In addition to the rental fees paid to the highland Juntas de Beneficencia for leases on the nationalized agricultural estates, two additional sources of financing for Beneficencia programs were (1) line items in the national budget and (2) various donations or bequests left for the purpose of advancing projects specified by the donors. See Ayora, *Informe*, xxii. In 1914, in the province of Pichincha, the institutions of Beneficencia included the Hospicio y Manicomio; the Lazareto (lepers' colony) de Pifo; the Hospital San Juan de Dios; the Maternidad lying-in clinic; orphanage facilities housed within the convents of San Carlos, Buen Pastor, and La Providencia; the Escuela Taller de Mujeres; the Escuela de Artes y Oficios; and Quito's new hospital in its planning stages (finally inaugurated in 1933 as the Hospital Eugenio Espejo). The products of nationalized haciendas were destined to support the Hospicio y Manicomio and the Hospital San Juan de Dios, there were funds from land sales that were deposited in an account for the new hospitals, and there were also a total of 116,000 sucres from the national budget dedicated to the support of these institutions (Peñaherrera, *Informe . . . 1914*, xxxvii). In 1915, with a renewal of rental leases on the nationalized estates on more advantageous terms for the Beneficencia, the previous income of 138,047.50 sucres was increased to 207,583.66 sucres,

of which 74,136 sucres were dedicated to sustaining the religious orders that "previously had usufruct of these properties," and the remaining rental income of 133,447.66 sucres was available for the support of urban social welfare institutions in the seven provinces of the north-central highlands. See Peñaherrera, *Informe . . . 1915*, xxxvi–xxxvii.

24. Díaz, *Informe*, xxxiii–xxxiv.

25. Ayora, *Informe*, xlvii.

26. Peñaherrera, *Informe . . . 1914*, xlvii.

27. The Ley de Sanidad can be found in Compañía Guía del Ecuador, *El Ecuador*, 239–40.

28. Pineo, "Misery and Death."

29. Ayora, *Informe*, l.

30. Becerra, "Informe," in Peñaherrera, *Informe . . . 1913*, 294.

31. Becerra, "Informe del Director de Sanidad," 510.

32. Becerra, "Informe," in Peñaherrera, *Informe . . . 1914*, 436.

33. There were indeed so few public health physicians that in early 1914 Miño had to be called away from Quito to head up the public health campaign in Esmeraldas on the north coast when serious outbreaks of malaria, yellow fever, and dysentery affected both the city population and the troops mobilized in the zone to fight the civil war. The director general found it indefensible that the service had to depend on the assistance of medical students or divert physicians from urgent duties elsewhere whenever there was an outbreak. The lack of medical facilities in most locations also caused elevated expenditures to transport supplies, a problem, he argued, that could be prevented if municipalities would establish small hospitals in the most important locales (Becerra, "Informe," in Peñaherrera, *Informe . . . 1914*, 431–32).

34. Becerra, "Informe del Director de Sanidad," 510.

35. Miño, "Informe," 441.

36. Becerra, "Informe del Director de Sanidad," 503.

37. See Peñaherrera, *Informe . . . 1916*, cx; and Becerra, "Informe del Director General de Sanidad Pública," 546.

38. For instance, monthly accounts (in LCE-1916, ASS/MNM) showed that in 1916 directly collected public health-related funeral taxes produced 3,825 sucres for the Quito subdirectorate that year, whereas less than 2,000 sucres had been collected through the tax farming system previously used.

39. Director general of Sanidad to the subdirector of Sanidad for Pichincha, Guayaquil, October 14, 1917, LCR-1917, ASS/MNM; secretary of the directorate of Sanidad to subdirector of Sanidad for Pichincha, Guayaquil, October 14, 1917, LCR-1917, ASS/MNM.

40. Director general of Sanidad to the subdirector of Sanidad for Pichincha, Guayaquil, February 17, 1918, LCR-1918-I, ASS/MNM.

41. While these financial constraints had a major impact, public health

activities were not singled out for neglect: these problems point us to larger issues affecting public administration in Ecuador. As economic historian Linda Rodríguez argues three decades ago, in an analysis that continues to be essential reading, the national budgeting process in Ecuador gave the executive branch little direct control over national finances since Congress pledged the majority of ordinary government revenue by statute to special programs. While in 1924 there was a proposal to develop a unified national budget, freeing up revenue streams to be able to dedicate them to projects determined to be of greatest importance, the national budgeting process was not overhauled until after the 1925 Revolución Juliana, when wide-ranging reforms to public administration processes were established. In addition to the problems generated by the budgeting structure, Rodríguez also demonstrates that frequently the actual revenues available for government projects and services fell considerably below the budgeted amounts (this was the case in twenty-three of the thirty fiscal years from 1896 to 1925). In unusual years where there was a surplus of actual over-budgeted revenue, the surfeit was invariably consumed by extraordinary expenditures. In the more common years where there was a deficit of actual revenue compared to what was budgeted, that deficit was usually increased further by unbudgeted expenditures. There was thus a considerable disconnect between what was budgeted to support a government agency and funds that actually flowed to it, the results of which can be seen clearly in the struggles to address public health threats. Rodríguez further shows that the figures for actual government revenues consistently included bank loans to the government, another issue of central concern at the time of the Revolución Juliana, which motivated considerable changes to public administration in the Revolution's aftermath (Rodríguez, *Search for Public Policy*).

42. Deler, *Ecuador: Del espacio*, 204.

43. Smith and Griffith, *Simply Institutional Ethnography*, 33–34.

44. Director general of Sanidad to the subdirector of Sanidad for Pichincha, Guayaquil, November 25, 1915, LCR-1915, ASS/MNM.

45. Smith and Griffith, *Simply Institutional Ethnography*, 31.

46. Tara A. Schwegler provides fascinating insight into how Mexican government officials cobbled together information and intuited signals pointing to possible policy shifts, something that was far from transparent to them even from their positions within the government bureaucracy ("Navigating the Illegible State").

47. Various documents mentioning Miño's positions outside the subdirectorate can be found in the ASS/MNM communications books for 1919 and 1920.

48. Director general of Sanidad to the subdirector of Sanidad for Pichincha, Guayaquil, March 27, 1914, LC-1914, ASS/MNM.

49. Municipal physician of Latacunga to the subdirector of Sanidad for Pichincha, Latacunga, March 18, 1916, LCR-1916, ASS/MNM.

50. Some suggestive parallels can be found in the challenges faced by operational meteorologists; see Fine, *Authors of the Storm*.

51. Miño, "Informe," 442.

52. Becerra, "Informe del Director de Sanidad," 505, 507.

53. Clark, *Gender, State, and Medicine*, 130–31.

54. See, for instance, governor of Chimborazo province to the director of Sanidad for the northern district, Riobamba, August 18, 1925, LCR-1925-II, ASS/MNM.

55. Director general of Sanidad to the municipal council president of Riobamba, Quito, April 6, 1926, LCE-1926, ASS/MNM.

56. The changing of the guard may have been facilitated by the fact that Wenceslao Pareja retired from the Sanidad effective April 1, 1926 and traveled to Europe for health reasons.

57. Suárez saw his work at the Universidad Central as his primary role, and he apparently took on leadership of the Sanidad on a transitory basis, according to at least two letters of resignation from the Sanidad role that he submitted in late December 1927 and June 1928 (in LCE-1927 and LCE-1928-I, ASS/MNM), which were not accepted. Dr. Alfonso Mosquera Narváez, who had assisted Suárez in the Sanidad directorate, replaced him as director general in late September 1928.

58. "Informe de la Delegación Especial de Sanidad de la Zona Austral al Ministro y Director General de Sanidad," Quito, August 20, 1926, LCR-Delegaciones Provinciales-1926/27, ASS/MNM.

59. The verbal discussion around the table at the conference is recorded in "Actas de la Primera Conferencia." More detailed written texts outlining the organizational structure of the various national public health services (which were circulated among colleagues at the conference) were also published in the *Boletín*—for instance, Suárez, "Organización Sanitaria."

60. The JBG continued to maintain its autonomous organization, and it was delegated similar functions as the two highland Juntas Centrales de Asistencia Pública, overseeing Asistencia activities in the coastal provinces as well as in Guayaquil.

61. "Actas," 231. Generally, information in this and the next paragraph is drawn from Actas, 229–32.

62. "Actas," 230.

63. "Informe de la Delegación Especial de Sanidad de la Zona Austral al Ministro y Director General de Sanidad," Quito, August 20, 1926, LCR-Delegaciones Provinciales-1926/27, ASS/MNM.

64. Director general of Sanidad to inspector general of Sanidad, Quito, February 15, 1932; director general of Sanidad to minister of government and Sanidad, Quito, February 16, 1932; director general of Sanidad to minister of government and Sanidad, Quito, February 19, 1932; all LCE-1932, ASS/MNM.

65. H. S. Cumming to inspector general of Sanidad, March 28, 1932; in-

spector general of Sanidad to director general of Sanidad, Quito, April 6, 1932; "Informe Anual del Inspector General de Salud Pública al Director General de Sanidad," Quito, May 25, 1932; all LCR-Servicio Interno e Informes-1932, ASS/MNM. Drs. Benjamín Mostajo and Atilio Macchiavello Varas, leaders of the anti-plague campaigns in Peru and Chile, were also appointed to similar traveling representative positions.

66. Several conversations over the years with Marujita Martínez de Suárez, Pablo Arturo Suárez's daughter-in-law, helped to round out my understanding of her father-in-law's career and personality. I appreciate how generous she was with her time.

67. Subdirector of Sanidad for Pichincha to director general of Sanidad, Quito, January 16, 1915, LCE-1915, ASS/MNM.

68. This discussion is influenced by anthropologist James Ferguson's study of the wide-ranging social and political implications of rendering problems technical in *Anti-Politics Machine.*

Chapter 3: Reaching In

Epigraph: "Informe Anual que el Subdirector de Sanidad de las Provincias de Pichincha, Imbabura y Carchi eleva al Ministerio del Ramo y a la Dirección de Sanidad de Guayaquil, 1919–1920," 8–9, LCE-1920, ASS/MNM.

1. Capello, *City at the Center*; and Kingman Garcés, *La ciudad.*

2. Kingman Garcés, *La ciudad*, 143.

3. Bustos Lozano, "Quito en la transición"; and Luna Tamayo, *Historia y conciencia popular.*

4. Goetschel, *Educación de las mujeres*; and Clark, *Gender, State, and Medicine.*

5. See for instance, among others, Luzuriaga Jaramillo, "Abastecimiento de agua." Carrión, Goetschel, and Sánchez, *Breve historia*, provides helpful details of timelines for the installation and extension of various municipal services.

6. Capello, *City at the Center*, 12; and Deler, *Ecuador: Del espacio*, 187–92.

7. Capello, *City at the Center*, 15, 88.

8. Capello, *City at the Centre*, 95. In 1897, the "Quito municipality celebrated the realization of its long-time goal by passing a flurry of new fines, duties, and other revenue-producing devices. These included sales taxes, other commercial levies, and increased rates on popular diversions such as theaters, pool halls, and other revenue-producing devices. Perhaps their most important new sources of income came from the restoration of control over municipal property, which had been the primary means for raising revenue prior to the mid-nineteenth century" (Capello, *City at the Centre*, 96).

9. Decreto supremo, dated May 19, 1906, cited in Luzuriaga Jaramillo, "Abastecimiento de agua," 38.

10. While the municipal council president was elected by and from among those elected to the municipal council, the mayor was directly elected by urban residents who were eligible to vote.

11. Capello, *City at the Center*, 104–5.

12. Capello, *City at the Centre*, 87.

13. See Kingman Garcés, *La ciudad*, 185–87, 192–93.

14. Kingman Garcés, *La ciudad*, 89. See also Durán, *Irrupción del sector.*

15. Bustos Lozano, "Notas."

16. See Kingman Garcés, *La ciudad*, 285, for a discussion of this study.

17. Kingman Garcés, *La ciudad*, 293.

18. Capello, *City at the Center*, 98–99; and Luzuriaga Jaramillo, "Abastecimiento de agua," 39.

19. Miño Grijalva, *Ferrocarril y modernización*, 34.

20. Capello comments on Andrade Marín's participation in the late 1880s discussion over the tram line, which involved disputes about the urban limits (*City at the Center*, 92). Kingman Garcés adds that, during his 1888 tenure as municipal council president, Andrade Marín advanced the renaming of city streets from ones associated with their function to names that evoked national civics (*La ciudad*, 206–7).

21. Capello, *City at the Center*, 98–99.

22. Subsequently, he served as president of the Cámara de Diputados in 1912, and as such served as interim executive power for several months. He turned over presidential power to Leonidas Plaza Gutiérrez later that year.

23. Municipal council president to general inspector of hygiene, Quito, July 2, 1908, LC-1908/9, ASS/MNM.

24. General inspector of hygiene for Quito to the municipal police chief, Quito, August 27, 1908, LC-1908/9, ASS/MNM.

25. General inspector of hygiene for Quito to the minister of the interior, Quito, September 12, 1908, LC-1908/9, ASS/MNM.

26. Capello, *City at the Center*, 41.

27. Subdirector of Sanidad to the director of Sanidad, Quito, June 5, 1909, LC-1908/9, ASS/MNM.

28. Subdirector of Sanidad to the director of Sanidad, Quito, June 5, 1909, LC-1908/9, ASS/MNM.

29. Municipal council president to the director of hygiene, Quito, May 31, 1913, LC-Oficina de Higiene Municipal-1913, ASS/MNM.

30. More often written as *huasicamas*, these servants were members of Indigenous peasant tenant (*huasipungo*) households who provided rotating labor in the landowner's urban home, along with diverse agricultural tasks at the rural estate, as part of the payment for access to a subsistence plot on the *hacienda*. This is a reminder of the racialized rural labor relationships that underwrote urban life among highland elites.

31. General inspector to the médico ayudante, Quito, April 24, 1913, LC-Oficina de Higiene Municipal-1913, ASS/MNM.

32. Manuel Jijón Bello to municipal council president of Quito, Quito, October 14, 1913, LC-Oficina de Higiene Municipal-1913, ASS/MNM.

33. Delegate of Sanidad to the minister of the interior and Sanidad, Quito, October 17, 1913, LC-1913, ASS/MNM.

34. The previous month, the acting governor had also contacted Miño about what he was doing to control venereal diseases (September 5) and about his actions to address high rates of infant mortality (September 24). See Clark, *Gender, State, and Medicine*, 54, 79.

35. Delegate of Sanidad for Pichincha to the political administrator of Quito canton, Quito, October 27, 1913, LC-1913, ASS/MNM.

36. The political administrator was among those who expected a great deal from the Sanidad, including in areas that did not fall under the organization's mandate. For instance, he requested that Miño organize a service of medical attention for children to help address infant and child mortality, an area that at the time clearly fell under the responsibility of the Junta de Beneficencia given its jurisdiction over curative medical institutions and social welfare (Clark, *Gender, State, and Medicine*, 54–55).

37. Printed broadsheet "Reglamento de Sanidad," effective August 1, 1913 and circulated for public information on August 18, 1913, LC-1913, ASS/MNM.

38. In May 1915, Miño developed a revised Reglamento for Quito based on his experience there since 1913, with changes in numbering of the Reglamentos but few changes in their spirit (Subdirector of Sanidad for Pichincha to the director general of Sanidad, Quito, May 6, 1915, LCE-1915, ASS/MNM).

39. A preliminary analysis of the domestic inspection program in Quito is offered in Clark, "La formación."

40. Both quotes are from Subdirector of Sanidad for Pichincha to police intendant general, Quito, April 3, 1914, LC-1914, ASS/MNM.

41. Another area where the responsibilities of Sanidad officials and police authorities were heavily negotiated and shifted over time was in prostitution control associated with venereal disease prophylaxis (see Clark, *Gender, State, and Medicine*, chap. 3).

42. Subdirector of Sanidad to the municipal council president, Quito, January 23, 1914, LC-1914, ASS/MNM.

43. Vice president of the municipal council to the subdirector of Sanidad, Quito, April 7, 1914, LC-1914, ASS/MNM.

44. Ordenanza del 10 de septiembre de 1888, cited in Luzuriaga Jaramillo, "Abastecimiento de agua," 42.

45. Petition from Luis Ávalos G. to the "Director de Higiene y Sanidad," Quito, undated, LC-1914, ASS/MNM.

46. Transcribed in Director general of public works to the subdirector of Sanidad, Quito, October 15, 1915, LCR-1915, ASS/MNM.

47. Subdirector of Sanidad to Doña Mercedes Ramírez v. de Vivanco, Quito, October 21, 1915, LCE-1915, ASS/MNM.

48. Transcribed in Minister of the interior to the subdirector of Sanidad, November 13, 1915, LCR-1915, ASS/MNM.

49. Subdirector of Sanidad to the minister of the interior, November 16, 1915, LCE-1915, ASS/MNM.

50. Cornejo Gómez, "Informe," in Ayora, *Informe . . . 1912*, 334.

51. Becerra, "Informe del Director General de Sanidad Pública," 506.

52. Becerra, "Informe del Director de Sanidad," 506.

53. "Informe Anual que el Subdirector de Sanidad de Pichincha eleva al Señor Ministro y al Señor Director del Ramo, 1917–1918," 2, LCE-1918, ASS/MNM.

54. Memorandum to the general police intendant from the subdirector of Sanidad regarding infraction of Abelardo Montalvo, Quito, November 19, 1914, LC-1914, ASS/MNM.

55. See *Boletín Sanitario de la Subdirección de Sanidad de Pichincha*, 1, no. 1 (Enero 1919): 1, filed in LCE-1919, ASS/MNM.

56. The list is appended to Municipal council president to subdirector of Sanidad, Quito, November 25, 1915, LCR-1915, ASS/MNM.

57. Mentioned in "Informe Anual que el Subdirector de Sanidad de Pichincha eleva al Ministro y al Director del Ramo, 1916–1917," 12, LCE-1917, ASS/MNM.

58. Decree of the municipal police chief, Quito, December 29, 1917, LCR-1917, ASS/MNM.

59. Municipal council president of Quito to the subdirector of Sanidad of Pichincha, Quito, November 18, 1918, LCR-1918-II, ASS/MNM.

60. Miño, "Informe," 9.

61. Orden de clausura temporal, Quito, July 11, 1918, LCE-1918, ASS/MNM.

62. None of this would have been possible without the construction of the railway between the port and the highland capital, which permitted the transportation of machinery and supplies over the cordillera, including the upgrading of the water supply system.

63. "Informe Anual que el Subdirector de Sanidad de las Provincias de Pichincha, Imbabura y Carchi eleva al Ministerio del Ramo y a la Dirección de Sanidad de Guayaquil, 1919–1920," LCE-1920, ASS/MNM.

64. Luzuriaga Jaramillo, "Abastecimiento de agua," 38.

65. Capello, *City at the Center*, 101–2.

66. Capello, *City at the Center*, 96–97.

Chapter 4: Reaching Out

1. The province had a larger geographical reach before the eastern portion that extended into the Amazonian region (what is now Pastaza province) was separated in 1920 (Ibarra, "Ambato," 234).

2. Figures presented in this paragraph are from Dirección Nacional de Estadística, *Ecuador en cifras*, 53–58.

3. Ambato's capital in circulation grew from 473,900 sucres to 1,013,100 sucres in these ten years (Ibarra, "Ambato," 267). Additional information in this paragraph is drawn from Orellana, *Guía comercial geográfica*, 99–102.

4. Delegate of Sanidad to the minister of the interior and Sanidad, Quito, December 11, 1913, LC-1913, ASS/MNM.

5. Delegate of Sanidad to the minister of the interior and Sanidad, Quito, December 11, 1913, LC-1913, ASS/MNM.

6. Request to issue this permission included in Subdirector of Sanidad to the minister of Sanidad, Quito, September 13, 1921, LCE-1921, ASS/MNM.

7. Director general of Sanidad to the municipal council president of Ambato, Quito, February 3, 1927, LCE-1927, ASS/MNM.

8. Both Lunemburg's comments and Suárez's response are included in Director general of Sanidad to the president of the Ambato municipal council, Quito, March 25, 1927, LCE-1927, ASS/MNM.

9. Engineer Noroña, general director of public works, to the president of the Ambato municipal council, Quito, March 31, 1927, LCR-Delegaciones Provinciales-1926/27, ASS/MNM.

10. This information comes from the enrollment records of the Facultad de Medicina, Universidad Central del Ecuador, consulted in the Archivo General de la Universidad Central (AGUC).

11. Compañía Guía del Ecuador, *El Ecuador*; and Dirección Nacional de Estadística, *Ecuador en cifras*.

12. Director general of Sanidad to the delegate of Sanidad for Tungurahua, Quito, January 25, 1928, LCE-1928-I, ASS/MNM.

13. Sanidad delegate for Tungurahua to the director general of Asistencia Pública, Ambato, September 19, 1929, LCR-Direcciones de Zona/Delegaciones Provinciales/Delegaciones Especiales/Inspectores ad Honorem-1929, ASS/MNM.

14. See Clark, *Gender, State, and Medicine*, chaps. 2 and 4.

15. Sanidad delegate for Tungurahua to the director general of Sanidad, Ambato, December 6, 1929, LCR-Direcciones de Zona/Delegaciones Provinciales/Delegaciones Especiales/Inspectores ad Honorem-1929, ASS/MNM.

16. Director general of Sanidad to the Sanidad delegate for Tungurahua, Quito, December 10, 1929, LCE-1929-II, ASS/MNM.

17. Director general of Asistencia Pública to director general of Sanidad,

Quito, December 11, 1929, LCR-Funcionarios Públicos e Instituciones-1929, ASS/MNM.

18. Director general of Sanidad to the minister of social welfare and Sanidad, Quito, December 19, 1929, LCE -1929-II, ASS/MNM.

19. Director general of Asistencia Pública to director general of Sanidad, Quito, December 19, 1929, LCR-Funcionarios Públicos e Instituciones-1929, ASS/MNM.

20. "Exposición hecha por el delegado de Sanidad al I. Concejo Municipal en sesión de enero 14 de 1929," LCR-Direcciones de Zona/Delegaciones Provinciales/Delegaciones Especiales/Inspectores ad Honorem-1929, ASS/MNM.

21. Capello, *City at the Center*, 105.

22. The maternal-infant health program is discussed in much more detail in Clark, *Gender, State, and Medicine*, chap. 4, including an expanded analysis of the conflicts outlined here. The midwives and nurses hired were trained in the Faculty of Medicine, and both groups struggled to distinguish themselves, in the public's eyes, from a range of other practitioners who intervened in birthing and patient care.

23. Consuelo Rueda to the director of Sanidad, Ambato, January 22, 1937, LCR-Comunicaciones Varias-1937, ASS/MNM.

24. Printed broadsheet "Al Público," Ambato, June 1935, LCR-Delegaciones Provinciales-1935, ASS/MNM.

25. Delegate of Sanidad for Tungurahua to the director of Sanidad, Ambato, January 11, 1937, LCR-Delegaciones Provinciales-1937, ASS/MNM.

26. While in 1930 there had been twice as many births attended by empirics than by professionals in Ambato, by September 1938 more than half of the births in the canton were being attended by a medical professional of some kind, including the Sanidad midwife (Clark, *Gender, State, and Medicine*, 130–32).

27. Delegate of Sanidad for Tungurahua to the director general of Sanidad, Ambato, June 26, 1936, LCR-Delegaciones Provinciales-1936, ASS/MNM.

28. Delegate of Sanidad for Tungurahua to the director of Sanidad for the central zone, Ambato, April 21, 1939, LCR-Delegaciones Provinciales-1939-I, ASS/MNM.

29. Consuelo Rueda to the delegate of Sanidad for Tungurahua, Ambato, September 5, 1940, LCR-Delegaciones Provinciales-1940-II, ASS/MNM.

30. Consuelo Rueda to the director of Sanidad for the central zone, Ambato, August 1, 1940, LCR-Delegaciones Provinciales-1940-II, ASS/MNM.

31. Indeed, low salaries did cause the Sanidad to lose medical professionals to other institutions in the late 1930s and early 1940s. Longtime Chimborazo provincial Sanidad delegate Alfonso Villagómez (pictured in the photo that opens this book) had just recently resigned from the Sanidad to take up the better-paid position leading the new provincial Caja del Seguro (Social Securi-

ty) medical service when he was struck down by pneumonic plague. Consuelo Rueda herself left the Ambato Sanidad delegation to take a similar Sanidad position in Machachi outside Quito in 1941 before very quickly moving on to a better-paid position with the municipal government there.

32. Delegate of Sanidad for Tungurahua to the director of Sanidad for the central zone, Ambato, November 11, 1940, LCR-Solicitudes-1940, ASS/MNM.

33. Delegate of Sanidad for Tungurahua to the director of Sanidad for the central zone, Ambato, December 21, 1938, LCR-Delegaciones Provinciales-1938-II, ASS/MNM.

34. Dirección Nacional de Estadística, *Ecuador en cifras*, 56.

35. The word *professional* indicated university training, so the midwives referred to are those who graduated from the Faculty of Medicine, not those who gained their expertise in other ways.

Chapter 5: Regulating Pharmacies and Professional Defense in Highland Ecuador

1. Ayudante encargado of the subdirectorate of Sanidad to the police intendant, Quito, March 16, 1914, LC-1914, ASS/MNM. The Sanidad needed to enlist the police to fine transgressors until the Sanidad comisario position was created in 1918, and they still called on police assistance afterwards when the comisario needed support to enforce orders.

2. See Director of Sanidad to the dean of the Facultad de Medicina at the Universidad Central, Quito, March 2, 1915, LCE-1915, ASS/MNM.

3. Clark, *Gender, State, and Medicine*, chaps. 4–5.

4. See Abbott, *System of Professions*.

5. Among other uses, the Sanidad also drew on their registry when they periodically received queries from importers of patent drugs in Guayaquil about whether specific practitioners who had requested samples of medications were licensed to practice medicine, which determined whether they were eligible to receive such samples. Many responses were in the negative. See, for instance, Query from S.B. Villacis (on behalf of US companies he represented) to director of Sanidad, Guayaquil, February 6, 1933, LCR-Asistencia Pública y Varias Comunicaciones-1933, ASS/MNM; and various exchanges with Bruckmann & Co, Guayaquil, such as January 5, 1937 (LCE-1937-I), April 28, 1938 (LCE-1938-I), July 26, 1939 (LCE-1939-II), and August 19, 1939 (LCR-Comunicaciones Varias-1939), all ASS/MNM.

6. By the early 1930s, the nómina was sufficiently complete to be published periodically as a pamphlet for ease of distribution (Dirección General de Sanidad, *Nómina*).

7. Circular No. 113 from the subdirector of Sanidad for Pichincha to the

representatives of Quito's pharmacies, Quito, May 9, 1921, LCE-1921, ASS/MNM.

8. Circular from the subdirector of Sanidad to the owners and pharmacists of Quito's pharmacies, Quito, November 27, 1924, LC-1924, ASS/MNM.

9. Carlos Miño might have had a particularly difficult time in persuading reluctant physicians to register their credentials with his office. In 1922 Miño was characterized as "a physician without significant connections" in the Faculty of Medicine (Orellana, *Guía comercial geográfica*, 112). The two directors general of Sanidad in the late 1920s had much closer relations with the university than Miño. Suárez was a professor at the university and went on to become its rector, and Alfonso Mosquera Narváez's older brother Aurelio was a prominent professor in the Faculty of Medicine and also served as both dean and rector. These closer ties may have facilitated the establishment of the professional registry in the Sanidad office in the period after 1925. By the 1940s the Sanidad felt confident that their registry was complete for all physicians who had graduated between 1900 and 1940 (Chief of the Sanidad pharmacy and professional practice office to the dean of the Faculty of Medicine at the Universidad Central, Quito, January 18, 1945, LCE-Jefatura de Farmacias-1944/45, ASS/MNM).

10. Subdirector of Sanidad to the minister of Sanidad, rector of the Universidad Central, dean of the Facultad de Medicina, and president of the Federación de Estudiantes, Quito, January 20, 1921, LCE-1921, ASS/MNM.

11. Rector of the Universidad Central to the subdirector of Sanidad, Quito, February 21, 1921, LCR-1921, ASS/MNM.

12. For a longer discussion of Carmela Granja's career, see Clark, *Gender, State, and Medicine*, 137–40.

13. Circular from the ayudante encargado del despacho del servicio de Sanidad to the owners and legal representatives of Quito's pharmacies, Quito, September 11, 1926, LCE-1926, ASS/MNM.

14. Secretary of the Universidad Central to the director general of Sanidad, Quito, November 14, 1927, LCR-Generales-1927, ASS/MNM; and Notification to Sr. Mackensie transcribed in Director of Sanidad to the secretary of the Universidad Central, Quito, November 16, 1927, LCE-1927, ASS/MNM.

15. Similarly, physicians were authorized to do odontological work—for instance in provincial hospitals, such as in Ibarra—but dentists were not authorized to practice medicine. Dentists did however benefit from the prestige of their association with medicine, rather than being identified with mechanical work.

16. Executive decree amending Article 1 of the Ley de Boticas y Droguerías, June 18, 1937; in Rosales Larrea, *Recopilación de leyes*, 414–15.

17. Dean of the Facultad de Medicina, Cirugía, Farmacia y Odontología of the Universidad Central to the director of Sanidad, Quito, March 16, 1929, LC-Epidemiología/Servicio Interno-1929, ASS/MNM.

18. The Sindicato Médico Ecuatoriano was established in Quito in March 1928; a few months earlier, in November 1927, the Círculo Médico Nacional was established in Guayaquil. Despite their names, these seemed to be more regional than national in scope. The Quito Sindicato was founded under the leadership of Dr. Aurelio Mosquera Narváez (elder brother of public health physician Alfonso Mosquera Narváez), who at the time was rector of the Universidad Central; he went on to become president of Ecuador in 1938–1939, though his term was cut short by his sudden death in office. The Sindicato built on an earlier meeting that Suárez hosted at his home in 1921 with other young physicians in the capital to discuss both professional defense and how physicians might contribute to addressing national medico-social problems. The Sindicato was transformed in 1933 into the Asociación Médica de Quito.

19. In their complaint, they also identified two private pharmacies operating without licensed pharmacists (*farmacéuticos titulados*). According to the director of Sanidad, however, these were not actually pharmacies where medications were prepared but rather agencies that sold patent medicines, or *agencias para la venta de productos patentados.*

20. Transcribed in Minister of social welfare and Sanidad to the director general of Sanidad, Quito, April 4, 1930, LCR-Ministerios del Estado-1930, ASS/MNM.

21. Director general of Sanidad to the minister of social welfare and Sanidad, Quito, April 8, 1930, LCE-1930-I, ASS/MNM.

22. See Clark, *Gender, State, and Medicine*, chaps. 2 and 5, for more information about the Hermanas' position administering Ecuadorian hospitals and social welfare institutions.

23. Martínez, *Memoria del Secretario*, xxiv–xxv. Luis A. Martínez was the uncle of Luis Joaquín Martínez (see chapter 4).

24. A few other female students did partial studies, including recently graduated midwife Consuela Rueda (see chapter 4). Rueda graduated from the midwifery program at the Universidad Central in 1903 and then in 1904 registered for the preparatory year of pharmacy studies. She went on to study for three additional years, and it is not clear from the archives why she did not pursue her final year. She emerges from the archival records of both the AGUC and, for a later time period, the ASS as a determined woman with a restive intellect, seeking economic security through her own work (perhaps as a response to having lost her father before her studies began, as the university enrollment records document). This was confirmed for me by her great niece, historian Sonia Fernández Rueda, when I discovered by chance their kin connection. Rueda figures prominently in Clark, *Gender, State, and Medicine*, chap. 4.

25. Among other intriguing information, university enrollment records held in the Archivo General de la Universidad Central point to an emerging network of female professionals who supported each other in their aspirations

to train for healthcare careers. In 1930, pharmacy student Angela Torres, aged twenty-seven and in her fourth year of studies, hosted a twenty-one-year-old first-year dentistry student, Blanca Rosa del Pino, who lived with her in Quito; both were from provincial cities and did not have extended family in Quito. Without an older student like Torres willing to take responsibility for her, it would have been difficult for a young single woman like del Pino to pursue her studies away from her family. See Clark, *Gender, State, and Medicine*, chaps. 4 and 5, for additional information about female students in the Facultad de Medicina who studied for a variety of medical and paramedical careers in the first half of the twentieth century.

26. Pharmacy students to the director general of Sanidad, Quito, March 2, 1932, LCR-Dirección de Sanidad-1931-I, ASS/MNM.

27. Rector of the Universidad Central to the director general of Sanidad, February 10, 1933, Quito, LCR-Ministerios y Varias Autoridades-1933, ASS/MNM.

28. Minister of government and social welfare to the director general of Sanidad, Quito, June 13, 1933, LC-Boticas y Higiene Municipal-1933, ASS/MNM.

29. Director general of Sanidad to the minister of government and Sanidad, Quito, June 14, 1933, LC-Boticas y Higiene Municipal-1933, ASS/MNM.

30. Director general of Sanidad to the minister of government and Sanidad, Quito, June 17, 1933, LCE-1933, ASS/MNM.

31. Minister of government and social welfare to the director general of Sanidad, Quito, July 4, 1933, LC-Boticas y Higiene Municipal-1933, ASS/MNM.

32. Director general of Sanidad to the minister of government and Sanidad, Quito, July 5, 1933, LCE-1933, ASS/MNM.

33. Director general of Sanidad to the director of the Junta Central de Asistencia Pública, Quito, July 11, 1933, LCE-1933, ASS/MNM.

34. Director general of Sanidad to the minister of government and Sanidad, Quito, January 24, 1934, LCE-1934-I, ASS/MNM.

35. Recently graduated pharmacist Braulio Montenegro to the director general of Sanidad, Quito, November 30, 1933, LCR-Asistencia Pública y Varias Comunicaciones-1933, ASS/MNM.

36. Botica Popular owner Elicio Flor to the Sanidad comisario, Quito, undated [1933], LC-Boticas y Higiene Municipal-1933, ASS/MNM.

37. Memo from the director general of Sanidad to the directors of Quito's four newspapers, Quito, January 22, 1934, LCE-1934-I, ASS/MNM.

38. Director general of Sanidad to the minister of government and Sanidad, Quito, June 16, 1934, LCE-1934-I, ASS/MNM.

39. Ley sobre el Comercio del Opio, October 13, 1916; in Rosales Larrea, *Recopilación de leyes*, 503–5.

40. Executive decree of November 28, 1922, LCR-1922, ASS/MNM.

41. Reforms to the Law on Trade in Opium, November 4, 1924; in Rosales Larrea, *Recopilación de leyes*, 505–8.

42. Director general of Sanidad to the minister of Sanidad, Quito, September 23, 1927, LCE-1927, ASS/MNM.

43. Referred to in Inspector general of Sanidad to the director general of Sanidad, Quito, December 30, 1931, LCR-Direcciones y Delegaciones Provinciales-1931, ASS/MNM.

44. Petition from pharmacy owners to the director general of Sanidad, Quito, undated, filed in LCR-Comisiones/Proyectos/etc.-1932, ASS/MNM.

45. Minutes of meeting of pharmacy owners, pharmacists, and director general of Sanidad, Quito, filed in LCR-Comisiones/Proyectos/etc.-1932, ASS/MNM.

46. Memo to Eduardo Ledesma de Janón, owner of Botica Pichincha, transcribing the report of the pharmacy inspection commission, Quito, June 16, 1939, LCE-1939-I, ASS/MNM.

47. Auxiliar to the director of Sanidad to the minister of social welfare and Sanidad, Quito, August 27, 1942, LCE-1942, ASS/MNM.

48. Chief of pharmacy inspection to the owner of the Botica Pichincha, Quito, April 30, 1945, LCE-Jefatura de Farmacias-1944/45, ASS/MNM.

49. Owner of the Botica Pichincha to the Sanidad section chief for pharmacies, Quito, April 30, 1945, LCR-Farmacias y Profesiones Médicas-1945, ASS/MNM.

50. Reformed Ley de Boticas y Droguerías, August 7, 1946; in Rosales Larrea, *Recopilación de leyes*, 417–20.

51. Circular from Departamento de propaganda médica, L.I.F.E., to physicians, Quito, April 21, 1941, LCR-Comunicaciones Varias-1941, ASS/MNM. In 2021, L.I.F.E. celebrated the eightieth anniversary of its founding.

52. Technical inspector of Sanidad for the central zone to chief of pharmacy inspection and professional practice (*ejercicio profesional*), Quito, February 26, 1945, LC-Farmacias y Profesiones Médicas-1945, ASS/MNM.

53. Chief of pharmacies and professional practice to general police intendant, Quito, July 4, 1945, LCE-Jefatura de Farmacias-1944/45, AAS/MNM.

54. A final category of stakeholders in the commercialization of medications—consumers—was largely absent from the documentation.

55. Painter, "Prosaic Geographies," 761.

Conclusions

1. "Informe Anual que el Subdirector de Sanidad de las Provincias de Pichincha, Imbabura y Carchi eleva al Ministerio del Ramo y a la Dirección de Sanidad de Guayaquil, 1919–1920," LCE-1920, ASS/MNM.

2. Cooper, *State of Health*, 6–9.

3. These questions also underlay my first book: Clark, *Redemptive Work*.

4. Stevenson, *Life beside Itself*, esp. chaps. 1–3.

5. Painter, "Prosaic Geographies," 753.

6. Krupa, "State by Proxy."

7. Carey, *Health in the Highlands*. His broad argument that the racialization of Indigenous people was harsher in Guatemala than in Ecuador is compatible with my findings about Ecuadorian social dynamics.

8. Historian Valeria Coronel offers a rich analysis of the interventions of labor inspectors from the Ministry of Social Welfare in agrarian disputes in the late 1920s and 1930s in "Revolution in Stages," chap. 7. Similarly, Pablo Ospina Peralta's analysis of these conflicts in part three of his book *La aleación inestable* is highly suggestive in this regard.

9. Sáenz Vera, "Campaña antipestosa intensiva."

10. A reliance on technical fixes over improvement of living conditions is discussed by Marcos Cueto and Steven Palmer as one element in their concept of the "culture of survival" characterizing official responses to epidemics in Latin America. See, for instance, their discussion of DDT use in malaria campaigns in *Medicine and Public Health*, 144–47, 261–62.

11. Krupa, "State by Proxy," 324.

12. This is a question that Ospina Peralta also explores, from a somewhat different angle, in *La aleación inestable*.

Bibliography

Archives

A note on archival sources: The principal archive used in this research, the ASS/MNM, is not formally cataloged. Instead, documents are bound together in volumes with labels such as *Libro de comunicaciones, 1914* (*Book of Communications, 1914*). As a result, I cite documents with the abbreviated name and year of the bound volume in which they were found (in the example above, LC-1914, ASS/MNM) and the position or name of the sender and the recipient, with the date and the location from which they were sent. Where there are separate volumes compiling communications received and those sent, I use the acronyms LCE for *Libro de comunicaciones enviadas* (*Book of Communications Sent*) and LCR for *Libro de comunicaciones recibidas* (*Book of Communications Received*). In cases where the year's communications are divided by semester, volume I or II is indicated after the year. In later years, there are often separate volumes for communications received from different offices, so where relevant this additional volume identifying information is included.

AGUC Archivo General de la Universidad Central del Ecuador, Quito
ASS/MNM Archivo del Servicio de Sanidad, Museo Nacional de Medicina, Quito

Primary and Secondary Sources

Abbott, Andrew. *The System of Professions: An Essay on the Division of Expert Labor.* Chicago: University of Chicago Press, 1988.

Abrams, Philip. "Notes on the Difficulty of Studying the State." *Journal of Historical Sociology* 1, no. 1 (March 1988): 58–89.

"Actas de la Primera Conferencia Panamericana de Directores Nacionales de Sanidad Pública de las Repúblicas Americanas." *Boletín de la Oficina Sanitaria Panamericana* 6, no. 3 (1927): 171–293.

Alfaro, Eloy. "Message of President Eloy Alfaro to the Ecuadorian Congress," October 20, 1908. In *Foreign Relations of the United States Diplomatic Papers, 1908: The American Republics*, translated and reproduced, no. 79, sec. 19-Ecuador, document 233, 281–82. Washington, DC: Government Printing Office, 1908.

Anderson, Benedict. *Imagined Communities: Reflections on the Origin and Spread of Nationalism*. London: Verso, 1983.

Archetti, Eduardo. *El mundo social y simbólico del cuy*. Quito: CEPLAES, 1992.

Arcos, Carlos, and Carlos Marchán. "Apuntes para una discusión sobre los cambios en la estructura agraria serrana." *Revista Ciencias Sociales* 2, no. 5 (1978): 13–51.

Arcos, Carlos. "El espíritu del progreso: Los hacendados en el Ecuador del 900." *Cultura* 19 (1984): 107–34.

Ayora, José María. *Informe que el Ministro de lo Interior, Policía, Obras Públicas, etc. presenta a la Nación en 1912*. Quito: Imprenta y Encuadernación Nacionales, 1912.

Becerra, León. "Informe de la Dirección del Servicio de Sanidad Pública del Ecuador." In Peñaherrera, *Informe . . . 1913*, 287–94. Quito: Imprenta y Encuadernación Nacionales, 1913.

Becerra, León. "Informe de la Dirección del Servicio de Sanidad Pública del Ecuador." Appendix to Peñaherrera, *Informe . . . 1914*, 429–38. Quito: Imprenta y Encuadernación Nacionales, 1914.

Becerra, León. "Informe del Director de Sanidad." In Peñaherrera, *Informe . . . 1915*, 503–10. Quito: Imprenta y Encuadernación Nacionales, 1915.

Becerra, León. "Informe del Director General de Sanidad Pública." Appendix to Peñaherrera, *Informe . . . 1916*, 536–48. Quito: Imprenta y Encuadernación Nacionales, 1916.

Becker, Marc. *Indians and Leftists in the Making of Ecuador's Modern Indigenous Movements*. Durham, NC: Duke University Press, 2008.

Bertherat, E. "Plague around the World, 2010–2015." *World Health Organization Weekly Epidemiological Record* 91, no. 8 (2016): 89–104.

Birn, Anne-Emanuelle. "Revolution, the Scatological Way: The Rockefeller Foundation's Hookworm Campaign in 1920s Mexico." In *Disease in the History of Modern Latin America: From Malaria to AIDS*, edited by Diego Armus, 158–82. Durham, NC: Duke University Press, 2003.

Bustos Lozano, Guillermo. "Notas sobre economía y sociedad en Quito y la Sierra centro norte durante las primeras décadas del siglo XX." *Quitumbe* 7 (1990): 101–17.

Bustos Lozano, Guillermo. "Quito en la transición: Actores colectivos e identidades culturales urbanas (1920–1950)." In *Enfoques y estudios históricos: Quito a través de la historia*, coordinated by Paúl Aguilar, 163–88. Quito: Municipio de Quito, Ministerio de Asuntos Exteriores de España, 1992.

Capello, Ernesto. *City at the Center of the World: Space, History, and Modernity in Quito*. Pittsburgh: University of Pittsburgh Press, 2011.

Carey, David, Jr. *Health in the Highlands: Indigenous Healing and Scientific Medicine in Guatemala and Ecuador*. Berkeley: University of California Press, 2023.

Carrión, Andrea, Ana María Goetschel, and Nancy Sánchez. *Breve historia de los servicios en la ciudad de Quito*. Coordinated by Mario Vásconez. Quito: CIUDAD, 1997.

CBC News. "Plague-Infected Squirrel Closes California Campgrounds." July 25, 2013. http://www.cbc.ca/news/health/story/2013/07/25/health-us-squirrel-plague.html.

Clark, A. Kim. "Indians, the State and Law: Public Works and the Struggle to Control Labor in Liberal Ecuador." *Journal of Historical Sociology* 7, no. 1 (1994): 49–72.

Clark, A. Kim. "La formación del estado ecuatoriano en el campo y la ciudad, 1895–1925." *Procesos* (Quito), no. 19 (2002/3): 117–30.

Clark, A. Kim. "New Arenas of State Action in Highland Ecuador: Public Health and State Formation, c. 1925–1950." In *State Theory and Andean Politics: New Approaches to the Study of Rule*, edited by Christopher Krupa and David Nugent, 126–41. Philadelphia: University of Pennsylvania Press, 2015.

Clark, A. Kim. "Race, 'Culture' and Mestizaje: The Statistical Construction of the Ecuadorian Nation, 1930–1950." *Journal of Historical Sociology* 11, no. 2 (1998): 185–211.

Clark, A. Kim. "Racial Ideologies and the Quest for National Development: Debating the Agrarian Problem in Ecuador (1930–1950)." *Journal of Latin American Studies* 30, no. 2 (1998), 373–93.

Clark, A. Kim. "The Language of Contention in Liberal Ecuador." In *Culture, Economy, Power: Anthropology as Critique, Anthropology as Praxis*, edited by Winnie Lem and Belinda Leach, 150–62. Albany: State University of New York Press, 2002.

Clark, A. Kim. *Gender, State, and Medicine in Highland Ecuador: Modernizing Women, Modernizing the State, 1895–1950*. Pittsburgh: University of Pittsburgh Press, 2012.

Clark, A. Kim. *The Redemptive Work: Railway and Nation in Ecuador, 1895–1930*. Wilmington: Scholarly Resources, 1998.

Clarke, John. "The Work of Governing." In *Governing Cultures: Anthropological Perspectives on Political Labor, Power, and Government*, edited by Kendra Coulter and William R. Schumann, 209–31. New York: Palgrave MacMillan, 2012.

Compañía Guía del Ecuador. *El Ecuador: Guía comercial, agrícola e industrial de la república*. Guayaquil: Talleres de Artes Gráficos de E. Rodenas, 1909.

Cooper, Amy. *State of Health: Pleasure and Politics in Venezuelan Health Care under Chávez*. Berkeley: University of California Press, 2019.

Córdova, Gonzalo S. *Informe del Ministro de lo Interior y Policía, Obras Públicas, etc. al Congreso Ordinario de 1903*. Quito: Imprenta Nacional, 1903.

Cornejo Gómez, L. "Informe del Sr. Director del Servicio de Sanidad Pública del Ecuador." In *Informe que el Ministro de lo Interior, Policía, Obras Públicas, etc., presenta a la Nación en 1912*, by José María Ayora, 330–39. Quito: Imprenta y Encuadernación Nacionales, 1912.

Cornejo Gómez, Luis Felipe. "Informe del Delegado del Ecuador a la V Conferencia Sanitaria Internacional de las Repúblicas Americanas." Appendix to *Informe que el Ministro de lo Interior, Policía, Obras Públicas, etc. presenta a la Nación en 1912*, by José María Ayora, 345–56. Quito: Imprenta y Encuadernación Nacionales, 1912.

Coronel, Adriana Valeria. "A Revolution in Stages: Subaltern Politics, Nation-State Formation, and the Origins of Social Rights in Ecuador, 1834–1943." PhD diss., New York University, 2011.

Coronel, Valeria. *La última guerra del Siglo de las Luces: Revolución Liberal y republicanismo popular en Ecuador.* Quito: FLACSO, 2022.

Corrigan, Philip, and Derek Sayer. *The Great Arch: English State Formation as Cultural Revolution*. New York: Basil Blackwell, 1985.

Cueto, Marcos, and Steven Palmer. *Medicine and Public Health in Latin America: A History*. New York: Cambridge University Press, 2015.

Cueto, Marcos. "Andean Biology in Peru: Scientific Styles on the Periphery." *Isis* 80, no. 4 (December 1989): 640–58.

Cueto, Marcos. *The Return of Epidemics: Health and Society in Peru during the Twentieth Century*. Aldershot, England: Ashgate, 2001.

Cueto, Marcos. *The Value of Health: A History of the Pan American Health Organization*. Washington: Pan American Health Organization, 2007.

Cumming, Hugh S. "Commercial and Sanitary Relations with the West Coasts of Mexico, Central and South America." *Public Health Reports* 18, no. 49 (December 4, 1903), 2129–30.

Cumming, Hugh S. "Cooperación internacional en sanidad: Su desenvolvimiento y estado actual; Algunas resultados de las modernas medidas preventivas." *Boletín de la Oficina Sanitaria Panamericana* 12, no. 12 (1933): 1191–203.

Cumming, Hugh S., et al. "Pan American Conference of Directors of Public Health." *Public Health Reports* 41, no. 46 (November 12, 1926): 2585–92.

Cunningham, Andrew. "Transforming Plague: The Laboratory and the Identity of Infectious Disease." In *The Laboratory Revolution in Medicine*, edited by Andrew Cunningham and Perry Williams, 209–44. Cambridge: Cambridge University Press, 1992.

Dawson, Thomas C. *The South American Republics: Peru, Chile, Bolivia, Ecuador,*

Venezuela, Colombia, Panama. Vol. 2 of *The South American Republics*. New York: G. P. Putnam's Sons, 1904.

De Lapierre, J. *Informe del Ministro de lo Interior y Policía, encargado de las carteras de Relaciones Exteriores, Culto, Instrucción Pública, Justicia, Beneficencia, Agricultura é Inmigración y Obras Públicas a la Convención Nacional de 1896–1897*. Quito: Imprenta Nacional, 1897.

De León, Perry M., and Archer Harman. "Lack of Quarantine Stations on the West Coast of South America." *Public Health Reports* 16, no. 13 (March 29, 1901): 613–4.

Deler, Jean-Paul. *Ecuador: Del espacio al estado nacional*. Quito: Banco Central, 1987.

Díaz, Octavio. *Informe que a la Nación presenta el Ministro de lo Interior, Policía, Beneficencia, Obras Públicas, etc. en el año 1910*. Quito: Imprenta y Encuadernación Nacionales, 1910.

Dirección General de Sanidad. *Nómina de médicos y cirujanos, dentistas, farmacéuticos y obstetrices, inscritos en Quito y Guayaquil*. Quito: Imprenta Nacional, 1932.

Dirección Nacional de Estadística. *Ecuador en cifras, 1938–1942*. Quito: Imprenta del Ministerio de Hacienda, 1944.

Drinot, Paulo. *The Allure of Labor: Workers, Race, and the Making of the Peruvian State*. Durham, NC: Duke University Press, 2011.

Durán, Cecilia. *Irrupción del sector burócrata en el estado ecuatoriano, 1925–1944*. Quito: Abya-Yala and PUCE, 2000.

Dyl, Joanna L. "The War on Rats versus the Right to Keep Chickens: Plague and the Paving of San Francisco, 1907–1908." In *The Nature of Cities*, edited by Andrew C. Isenberg, 38–61. Rochester, NY: University of Rochester Press, 2006.

Echenberg, Myron. *Plague Ports: The Global Urban Impact of Bubonic Plague, 1894–1901*. New York: New York University Press, 2007.

"Ecuador: Health and Sanitary Condition of Guayaquil and Vicinity; Yellow Fever Epidemics." *Public Health Reports* 19, no. 19 (May 6, 1904): 861–81.

"Ecuador: Report from Quito; Plague Officially Recognized at Guayaquil—Precautionary Measures To Be Taken at Quito." *Public Health Reports* 23, no. 14 (April 3, 1908): 425.

"Ecuador: Reports from Guayaquil; Mortality among Rats—Plague Not Officially Announced; Yellow Fever at Guayaquil and Huigra." *Public Health Reports* 23, no. 10 (March 6, 1908): 284–5.

"El control de las enfermedades transmisibles: Informe presentado por la Comisión de la Asociación de Sanidad Pública Americana sobre Reglamentos Modelos, que fue nombrado en octubre de 1916." *Boletín de la Oficina Sanitaria Panamericana* 6, no. 4 (1927): 301–45.

Eskey, C. R. "Chief Etiological Factors of Plague in Ecuador and the Anti-plague Campaign: I. Chief Etiological Factors." *Public Health Reports* 45, no. 36 (September 5, 1930): 2077–115.

Evans, Nicholas H. A. "Blaming the Rat? Accounting for Plague in Colonial Indian Medicine." *Medicine Anthropology Theory* 5, no. 3 (2018): 15–42.

Farmer, Paul. *AIDS and Accusation: Haiti and the Geography of Blame*. Berkeley: University of California Press, 1992.

Farmer, Paul. *Fevers, Feuds, and Diamonds: Ebola and the Ravages of History*. New York: Farrar, Straus and Giroux, 2020.

Ferguson, James, and Akhil Gupta. "Spatializing States: Toward an Ethnography of Neoliberal Governmentality." *American Ethnologist* 29, no. 4 (2002): 981–1002.

Ferguson, James. *The Anti-Politics Machine: "Development," Depoliticization, and Bureaucratic Power in Lesotho*. New York: Cambridge University Press, 1990.

Fine, Gary Alan. *Authors of the Storm: Meteorologists and the Culture of Prediction*. Chicago: University of Chicago Press, 2007.

Gade, Daniel W. *Nature and Culture in the Andes*. Madison: University of Wisconsin Press, 1999.

Gluckman, Max. "Analysis of a Social Situation in Modern Zululand (Part 1)." *Bantu Studies* 14, no. 1 (1940): 1–30.

Goetschel, Ana María. *Educación de las mujeres, maestras y esferas públicas: Quito en la primera mitad del siglo XX*. Quito: Facultad Latinoamericana de Ciencias Sociales and Abya-Yala, 2007.

Gramsci, Antonio. "Notes on Italian History." In *Selections from the Prison Notebooks*, edited and translated by Quintin Hoare and Geoffrey Nowell Smith, 52–120. New York: International Publishers, 1971.

Grandin, Greg. *The Blood of Guatemala: A History of Race and Nation*. Durham, NC: Duke University Press, 2000.

Green, Monica H. "The Four Black Deaths." *American Historical Review* 125, no. 5 (2020): 1601–31.

"Guayaquil inscrito como puerto limpio de clase A." *Boletín de la Oficina Sanitaria Panamericana* 19, no. 5 (1940): 439.

"Guayaquil, puerto limpio de clase A." *Boletín de la Oficina Sanitaria Panamericana* 9, no. 12 (1930): 1420–23.

Guerrero, Andrés. "Una imagen ventrílocua: El discurso liberal de la 'desgraciada raza indígena.'" In *Imágenes e imagineros: Representaciones de los indígenas ecuatorianos, siglos XIX y XX*, edited by Blanca Muratorio, 197–252. Quito: FLACSO, 1994.

Ibarra, Hernán. "Ambato: Las ciudades y pueblos de la sierra central ecuatoriana (1800–1930)." In *Ciudades de los Andes: Visión histórica y contemporánea*, edited by Eduardo Kingman Garcés, 223–79. Quito: IFEA and CIUDAD, 1992.

Ibarra, Hernán. *Indios y cholos: Orígenes de la clase trabajadora ecuatoriana*. Quito: Editorial El Conejo, 1992.

Joseph, Gilbert M., and Daniel Nugent, eds. *Everyday Forms of State Formation: Revolution and the Negotiation of Rule in Modern Mexico*. Durham, NC: Duke University Press, 1994.

Keck, Frédéric, and Christos Lynteris. "Zoonosis: Prospects and Challenges for Medical Anthropology." *Medicine Anthropology Theory* 5, no. 3 (2018): 1–14.

Kelly, Ann H., Frédéric Keck, and Christos Lynteris, eds. *The Anthropology of Epidemics*. New York: Routledge, 2019.

Kingman Garcés, Eduardo. *La ciudad y los otros: Quito 1860–1940; Higienismo, ornato y policía*. Quito: FLACSO and Universidad Rovira e Virgili, 2006.

Krupa, Christopher, and David Nugent, eds. *State Theory and Andean Politics: New Approaches to the Study of Rule*. Philadelphia: University of Pennsylvania Press, 2015.

Krupa, Christopher. "State by Proxy: Privatized Government in the Andes." *Comparative Studies in Society and History* 52, no. 2 (2010): 319–50.

"La pandemia actual de la peste." *Boletín de la Oficina Sanitaria Panamericana* 4, no. 1 (1925): 30–34.

Lloyd, B. J. "Plague: Past, Present and Future." *Journal of the American Medical Association* 85, no. 10 (September 5, 1925): 729–33.

Loewenfeld, Eva. "The Guayaquil and Quito Railway, Ecuador." *Southwestern Social Science Quarterly* 27, no. 1 (1946): 68–93.

Long, John D. "Bubonic Plague on the West Coast of South America in 1934." *Public Health Reports* 50, no. 29 (July 19, 1935): 923–32.

Long, John D. "Choice of Rat Poison in Antiplague Work: Rat Poisons Used by the National Antiplague Services of Ecuador, Peru, Chile, and the Argentine Republic." *Public Health Reports* 51, no. 18 (May 1, 1936): 551–4.

Long, John D. "La campaña antipestosa en Guayaquil." *Boletín de la Oficina Sanitaria Panamericana* 9, no. 8 (1930): 921–30.

Luna Tamayo, Milton. *Historia y conciencia popular: El artesanado en Quito, economía, organización y vida cotidiana, 1890–1930*. Quito: Corporación Editora Nacional, 1989.

Luzuriaga Jaramillo, Sofía. "Abastecimiento de agua y políticas de saneamiento en Quito, 1880–1930." *Procesos* 32 (2010): 31–52.

Lynteris, Christos and Branwyn Poleykett. "The Anthropology of Epidemic Control: Technologies and Materialities." *Medical Anthropology* 37, no. 6 (2018): 433–41.

Maiguashca, Juan, and Liisa North. "Orígenes y significado del velasquismo: Lucha de clases y participación política en el Ecuador, 1920–1972." In *La cuestión regional y el poder*, edited by Rafael Quintero, 89–159. Vol. 29 of *Biblioteca de ciencias sociales*. Quito: Corporación Editora Nacional, 1991.

Maiguashca, Juan. "Los sectores subalternos en los años 30 y el aparecimiento del velasquismo." In *Las crisis en el Ecuador: Los treinta y ochenta*, edited by Rosemary Thorp, 79–94. Vol. 33 of *Biblioteca de ciencias sociales*. Quito: Corporación Editora Nacional, 1991.

Mallon, Florencia E. *Peasant and Nation: The Making of Postcolonial Mexico and Peru*. Berkeley: University of California Press, 1995.

Marchán Romero, Carlos. "La crisis de los años treinta: Diferenciación social de sus efectos económicos." In *Las crisis en el Ecuador: Los treinta y ochenta*, edited by Rosemary Thorp, 31–60. Vol. 33 of *Biblioteca de ciencias sociales*. Quito: Corporación Editora Nacional, 1991.

Martínez Vinueza, Juan J. "Peste eruptiva (viruela pestosa) y angina pestosa: Formas raras de la peste." *Boletín de la Oficina Sanitaria Panamericana* 9, no. 10 (1930): 1189–95.

Martínez, Luis A. *Memoria del Secretario de Instrucción Pública, Correos y Telégrafos, etc. al Congreso Ordinario de 1905*. Quito: Tipografía de la Escuela de Artes y Oficios, 1905.

Mena Villamar, Claudio. *Ecuador a comienzos de siglo*. Quito: Abya-Yala and Letranueva, 1995.

Milton, Cynthia. *The Many Meanings of Poverty: Colonialism, Social Compacts, and Assistance in Eighteenth-Century Ecuador*. Stanford, CA: Stanford University Press, 2007.

Miño Grijalva, Wilson. *Ferrocarril y modernización en Quito: Un cambio dramático entre 1905 y 1922*. Quito: Universidad Andina Simón Bolívar, 2018.

Miño, Carlos A. "Informe de la Subdirección de Sanidad de la provincia de Pichincha al Ministro de Sanidad y al Director del Servicio de Sanidad Pública." Appendix to Peñaherrera, *Informe . . . 1914*, 439–46. Quito: Imprenta y Encuadernación Nacionales, 1914.

Miño, Carlos A. *La peste bubónica en el Ecuador: Factores etiológicos, formas clínicas y erradicación*. Quito: Imprenta Nacional, 1933.

Mitchell, Timothy. "The Limits of the State: Beyond Statist Approaches and Their Critics." *American Political Science Review* 85, no. 1 (1991): 77–96.

Moll, Aristides A., and Shirley Baughman O'Leary. "Plague in the Americas: An Historical and Quasi-Epidemiological Survey (Part 1)." *Boletín de la Oficina Sanitaria Panamericana* 19, no. 5 (1940): 451–61.

Moll, Aristides A., and Shirley Baughman O'Leary. "Plague in the Americas: An Historical and Quasi-Epidemiological Survey (Part 12)." *Boletín de la Oficina Sanitaria Panamericana* 20, no. 4 (1941): 365–74.

Moncayo, Abelardo. *Informe del Ministro de lo Interior y Policía, Beneficencia, etc. al Congreso Ordinario de 1898*. Quito: Imprenta Nacional, 1898.

Moncayo, Abelardo. *Informe del Ministro de lo Interior y Policía, Beneficencia, etc. al Congreso de 1899*. Quito: Imprenta Nacional, 1899.

Mordechai, Lee, and Merle Eisenberg. "Rejecting Catastrophe: The Case of the Justinianic Plague." *Past and Present* 244, no. 1 (2019): 3–50.

Murdock, John R. "Pneumonic Plague in Ecuador during 1939." *Public Health Reports* 55, no. 47 (November 22, 1940): 2172–8.

New York Times. "Guayaquil Has Lost Place as 'Pest Hole.'" August 30, 1931, E8.

O'Connor, Erin. *Gender, Indian, Nation: The Contradictions of Making Ecuador, 1830–1925*. Tucson: University of Arizona Press, 2007.

Orellana, J. Gonzalo. *Guía comercial geográfica: Comprende las provincias de Pichincha, León, Tungurahua, Chimborazo y Guayas*. Guayaquil: Imprenta de la Escuela de Artes y Oficios de la Sociedad Filantrópica del Guayas, 1922.

Ospina Peralta, Pablo. *La aleación inestable: Origen y consolidación de un estado transformista; Ecuador, 1920–1960*. Buenos Aires: Teseo; Quito: Universidad Andina Simón Bolívar, 2020.

Painter, Joe. "Prosaic Geographies of Stateness." *Political Geography* 25, no. 7 (2006): 752–74.

Palmer, Steven. *From Popular Medicine to Medical Populism: Doctors, Healers, and Public Power in Costa Rica, 1800–1940*. Durham, NC: Duke University Press, 2003.

Palmer, Steven. *Launching Global Health: The Caribbean Odyssey of the Rockefeller Foundation*. Ann Arbor: University of Michigan Press, 2010.

"Panama: Plague Conditions on West Coast of South America a Menace to Panama; Necessity for Increased Quarantine Facilities." *Public Health Reports* 19, no. 27 (July 1, 1904): 1339–40.

Parks, Lois F., and Gustave A. Nuermberger. "The Sanitation of Guayaquil." *Hispanic American Historical Review* 23, no. 2 (1943): 197–221.

Paz y Miño Cepeda, Juan José. *Revolución Juliana: Nación, ejército y bancocracia*. 2nd ed. Quito: Abya-Yala, 2000.

Peñaherrera, Modesto A. *Informe que Modesto A. Peñaherrera, Ministro de lo Interior, Municipalidades, Policía, Obras Públicas, etc., presenta a la Nación en 1913*. Quito: Imprenta y Encuadernación Nacionales, 1913.

Peñaherrera, Modesto A. *Informe que Modesto A. Peñaherrera, Ministro de lo Interior, Municipalidades, Policía, Obras Públicas, etc., presenta a la Nación en 1914*. Quito: Imprenta y Encuadernación Nacionales, 1914.

Peñaherrera, Modesto A. *Informe que Modesto A. Peñaherrera, Ministro de lo Interior, Municipalidades, Policía, Obras Públicas, etc., presenta a la Nación en 1915*. Quito: Imprenta y Encuadernación Nacionales, 1915.

Peñaherrera, Modesto A. *Informe que Modesto A. Peñaherrera, Ministro de lo Interior, Municipalidades, Policía, Obras Públicas, etc., presenta a la Nación en 1916*. Quito: Imprenta y Encuadernación Nacionales, 1916.

Pineo, Ronn F. "Misery and Death in the Pearl of the Pacific: Health Care in Guayaquil, Ecuador, 1870–1925." *Hispanic American Historical Review* 70, no. 4 (1990): 609–37.

Pineo, Ronn F. *Social and Economic Reform in Ecuador: Life and Work in Guayaquil.* Gainesville: University Press of Florida, 1996.

Pollitzer, Robert. *Plague.* Geneva: World Health Organization, 1954.

Prieto, Mercedes. *Liberalismo y temor: Imaginando los sujetos indígenas en el Ecuador postcolonial, 1895–1950.* Quito: FLACSO, 2004.

Puga, Amalio. *Informe del Ministerio de lo Interior, Policía, Beneficencia, Obras Públicas, etc. a la Nación en 1908.* Quito: Imprenta Nacional, 1908.

Reyes V., Alejandro. *Informe del Ministerio de lo Interior, Policía, Beneficencia, Obras Públicas, etc. a la Nación en 1909.* Quito: Imprenta Nacional, 1909.

Rodas Chaves, Germán. *Pensamiento médico: El liberalismo radical y la Revolución Juliana; Trazos de la figura de Isidro Ayora.* Quito: Universidad Andina Simón Bolívar, 2017.

Rodríguez, Linda Alexander. *The Search for Public Policy: Regional Politics and Government Finances in Ecuador, 1830–1940.* Berkeley: University of California Press, 1985.

Rojas M., Milton, and Gaitán Villavicencio. *El proceso urbano de Guayaquil, 1870–1980.* Guayaquil: Instituto Latinoamericano de Investigaciones Sociales (ILDIS) and Centro de Estudios Regionales de Guayaquil (CER-G), 1988.

Rosales Larrea, Adriano. *Recopilación de leyes y reglamentos de sanidad del Ecuador.* Quito: Editorial Fray Jodoco Ricke, 1961.

Sáenz Vera, Cornelio. "Brote de peste en la provincia de Riobamba, Ecuador." *Boletín de la Oficina Sanitaria Panamericana* 19, no. 1 (1940): 40–43.

Sáenz Vera, Cornelio. "Campaña antipestosa intensiva en la provincia del Chimborazo (Ecuador)." *Boletín de la Oficina Sanitaria Panamericana* 22, no. 10 (1943): 873–82.

Schwegler, Tara A. "Navigating the Illegible State: The Political Labor of Government in Mexico." In *Governing Cultures: Anthropological Perspectives on Political Labor, Power, and Government*, edited by Kendra Coulter and William R. Schumann, 21–46. New York: Palgrave MacMillan, 2012.

"Second General International Sanitary Convention of the American Republics: Sanitary Convention Ad Referendum." *Public Health Reports* 22, no. 5 (February 1, 1907): 93–101.

Slack, Paul. "Perceptions of Plague in Eighteenth-Century Europe." *Economic History Review* 75, no. 1 (February 2022): 138–56.

Slack, Paul. *Plague: A Very Short Introduction.* Oxford: Oxford University Press, 2012.

Smith, Dorothy E. *Institutional Ethnography: A Sociology for People.* Lanham, MD: AltaMira Press, 2005.

Smith, Dorothy E., and Alison I. Griffith. *Simply Institutional Ethnography: Creating a Sociology for People.* Toronto: University of Toronto Press, 2022.

Sodikoff, Genese Marie. "The Multispecies Infrastructure of Zoonosis." In Kelly, Keck, and Lynteris, *Anthropology of Epidemics*, 102–20. New York: Routledge, 2019.

Stevenson, Lisa. *Life beside Itself: Imagining Care in the Canadian Arctic*. Oakland: University of California Press, 2014.

Suárez, Pablo Arturo. "Organización Sanitaria del Ecuador." *Boletín de la Oficina Sanitaria Panamericana* 6, no. 2 (1927): 108–19.

Suárez, Pablo Arturo. *Contribución al estudio de las realidades entre las clases obreras y campesinas*. Quito: Imprenta de la Universidad Central, 1934.

Torre, Patricia de la. *La Junta de Beneficencia de Guayaquil: Lo privado y local en el estado ecuatoriano*. Quito: Abya-Yala, 1999.

Trouillot, Michel-Rolph. "The Anthropology of the State in the Age of Globalization: Close Encounters of the Deceptive Kind." *Current Anthropology* 42, no. 1 (2001): 125–38.

Valverde, Miguel. *Informe del Ministro de lo Interior y Policía, Obras Públicas, etc. al Congreso Ordinario de 1902*. Quito: Imprenta Nacional, 1902.

Williams, Derek. "Assembling the 'Empire of Morality': State Building Strategies in Catholic Ecuador, 1861–1875." *Journal of Historical Sociology* 14, no. 2 (2001): 149–74.

Wolf, Teodoro. *Geografía y geología del Ecuado*. Quito: Casa de la Cultura Ecuatoriana, 1975. First published 1892 by F. A. Brockhaus.

World Health Organization. "Health Topics: Plague." Accessed March 14, 2021. https://www.who.int/health-topics/plague#tab=tab_1.

"World Prevalence of Human Plague in 1923." *Public Health Reports* 40, no. 5 (January 30, 1925): 191–202.

Index

Note: References in *italics* refer to figures and tables.